The International Library of Bioethics

Founding Editors

David N. Weisstub
Thomasine Kimbrough Kushner

Volume 99

The *International Library of Bioethics* – formerly known as the International Library of Ethics, Law and the New Medicine comprises volumes with an international and interdisciplinary focus on foundational and applied issues in bioethics. With this renewal of a successful series we aim to meet the challenge of our time: how to direct biotechnology to human and other living things' ends, how to deal with changed values in the areas of religion, society, and culture, and how to formulate a new way of thinking, a new bioethics.

The *International Library of Bioethics* focuses on the role of bioethics against the background of increasing globalization and interdependency of the world's cultures and governments, with mutual influencing occurring throughout the world in all fields. The series will continue to focus on perennial issues of aging, mental health, preventive medicine, medical research issues, end of life, biolaw, and other areas of bioethics, whilst expanding into other current and future topics.

We welcome book proposals representing the broad interest of this series' inter-disciplinary and international focus. We especially encourage proposals addressing aspects of changes in biological and medical research and clinical health care, health policy, medical and biotechnology, and other applied ethical areas involving living things, with an emphasis on those interventions and alterations that force us to re-examine foundational issues.

Frida Simonstein

Womb Politics: A Short History of the Future of Human Reproduction

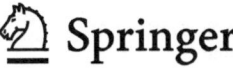 Springer

Frida Simonstein
School of Public Health
Ben-Gurion University of the Negev
Beersheba, Israel

ISSN 2662-9186   ISSN 2662-9194 (electronic)
The International Library of Bioethics
ISBN 978-3-031-11653-7   ISBN 978-3-031-11654-4 (eBook)
https://doi.org/10.1007/978-3-031-11654-4

This Springer imprint is published by the registered company Springer Nature Switzerland AG
The registered company address is: Gewerbestrasse 11, 6330 Cham, Switzerland

In memory of Yochanan Simonstein

Acknowledgments

It may take more than nine months—the human gestation period—for a tiny idea to grow and become a full-fledged book. So first, I want to thank John Harris, who—unwittingly—put the tiny idea in my mind almost twenty years ago, when I realized that in an enhancement scenario, women are taken for granted. And to Matty Häyry, who, while speaking at an ESPMH conference, said that having children is immoral. For me, hailing from a paternalistic country where childbirth is a must for women—and IVF their greatest savior—Häyry's provocative idea was shocking and eye-opening. I am thankful also to Daniel Callahan for his support for my research on ectogenesis and the artificial womb at the Hastings Center; to Miriam Hirschfeld, who made it possible for me to spend a summer at the WHO; to Shimon Glick, who shared his thoughts with me on women's desire to become mothers; to Ariel Ravel and Johnny Younis, who (anonymously) opened the archives of their IVF clinics; to Ekaterina Balabanova, who collaborated with me in IVF research in a developing country; to Ada Geva, who kindly introduced me to infertile women in the Bible; our discussions, over coffee, about their miraculous pregnancies were delightful; and to Michal Mashiach, who prepared the statistics analyses in Chaps. 8 and 11 and with whom I shared many hours of arduous work and friendship. I am thankful also to my dearest friends, Lily Sade and the late Shula Gilboa, who discussed some of the ideas in this book with me; to Sarah Veeder, my language editor, who patiently translated my English into English; and to Floor Oosting, the editor at Springer, who believed in this project. Finally, but not least, I am grateful to my family, to my children, and especially to their father, my life partner, who was always supportive of my academic choices and with whom I endlessly discussed the ideas for this book. He died before the idea became real. I am dedicating this book to his memory.

Contents

Abbreviations

ART	Artificial reproductive technology
AW	Artificial womb
CDC	Centers of Disease Control
COH	Controlled ovarian hyperstimulation
COS	Controlled ovarian stimulation
ELBW	Extremely low birth weight
FSH	Follicle stimulant hormone
FTE	Full-time employment
GnRh	Gonadotropin-releasing hormone
hCG	Human chorionic gonadotropin
HFEA	Human Fertilization and Embryology Authority
HIV	Human immunodeficiency virus
ICSI	Intracytoplasmic sperm injection
IDF	Israeli Defense Force
IUD	Intrauterine device
IVF	In vitro fertilization
LH	Luteinizing hormone
MoH	Ministry of Health
NGO	Non-Governmental Organization
NHI	National Health Insurance
NICU	Neonatal Intensive Care Unit
NIH	National Institute of Health
OHSS	Ovarian hyperstimulation syndrome
PGD	Pre-implantation genetic diagnosis
PPB	Principle of procreative beneficence
PTSD	Post-traumatic stress disorder
PVS	Persistent vegetative state
WHO	World Health Organization
ZIFT	Zygote intra-fallopian transfer

Chapter 1
Introduction

Whenever people ask me what I am writing about, their reactions to my answer are invariably along the lines of: "What? What does politics have to do with the womb?" Or, with a certain awkwardness: "What? Politics meddles with the womb as well?" Most women (and men) appear to be unaware of the political status of our reproductive organ. This, perhaps, should not come as such a surprise, as we are taught gender roles since the day we are born. Isn't having babies what women are supposed and want to do? Isn't reproduction a private matter? How can it be a political issue? But it is.

Womb Politics may be reminiscent of the term Gender Politics, which is defined as the assumptions underlying expectations regarding gender difference in a society [and] an ideology based on such assumptions. This notion originated in the Gender Studies field in the 1970s. Gender Politics has been used to argue that issues such as spousal abuse or reproductive rights, considered private as opposed to public issues, "should be politicized" and considered as matters of public concern.[1] However, I argue throughout this book that reproduction also considered a "private" issue is highly politicized and has been a matter of public concern since biblical times and possibly, before.

Politics is a contested concept, but one of its definitions is "the exercise of power," which applies to the context of this book. According to the political scientist Robert A. Dahl, "power" is the influence over the actions of others: "A has power over B to the extent that he can get B to do something that B would not otherwise do" (Dahl 1957). Nonetheless, Dahl's critics argued that his definition did not capture other important dimensions of power, "such as the capacity of an actor to shape the norms and values held by others."[2] In the context of this book, both definitions of power

---

[1] https://www.open.edu/openlearn/society-politics-law/what-politics. Accessed 3.5.2021.

[2] https://www.britannica.com/biography/Robert-A-Dahl#ref1178984. P. 202–3. Accessed 3.6.2021.

F. Simonstein, *Womb Politics: A Short History of the Future of Human Reproduction*,
The International Library of Bioethics 99,
https://doi.org/10.1007/978-3-031-11654-4_11

are adequate. Nevertheless, the definition that may best serve the notion of Womb
Politics is that of Adrian Leftwich:

> In politics… power is usually thought of as…the ability to influence the behavior of others
> in a manner not of their choosing. This implies having 'power over' people (Adrian 2004).

Womb Politics entails having power over the womb which, by Leftwich's
definition, implies having power over those who possess one.

The issues dealt with in this book are not new. The uniqueness of this volume
is that it brings together areas of study and disciplines that have traditionally been
discussed separately. My aim is to present a bigger picture of the political powers
that actually rule over women's reproductive tasks. Although feminism has tried to
separate women from their wombs, rightly contending that women are much more
than reproductive vessels, a more comprehensive picture of the historical, present,
and future demands over women's reproductive organ is needed. A broader picture
may help women (and men) to gain an informed understanding of their reproductive
decisions and may contribute to improving women's lives.

This volume examines gender, demographic needs, requests, and commandments
that have ruled over the womb since biblical times. It addresses the advent of the
pill in the 1960s and the struggle for lawful abortions that is still ongoing in the
twenty-first century. It looks at assisted reproduction technologies (ARTS) with
in vitro fertilization (IVF) that appeared in the twentieth century and examines
the arrival of reprogenetics in the twenty-first century to "enhance" future generations genetically, a procedure that would eventually require all women to undergo
IVF. Finally, this book explores the advent of the artificial womb (AW). Bioethi-
cists/lawyers/historians/futurists may find this book useful, but it may be of interest
also to the general public.

Chapter 2 examines notions of gender and its biases. It explores patriarchy and
the theories that might explain its development in all human societies. It looks at
the advent of feminism and its discontents. This chapter concludes by exploring
motherhood and the notions of "womanhood" that may still be holding women back.

According to Yuval Noah Harari, throughout history, no matter how a society
defined "man" or "woman," it has always been preferable to be a man (Harari 2014).
Patriarchal societies educate men to think and act in masculine ways and women to
think and act in feminine ways, punishing anyone who dares cross those boundaries
(Criado Perez 2019). However, as Harari notes, those who conform are not rewarded
equally:

> Qualities considered masculine are more valued than those considered feminine, and
> members of a society who personify the feminine ideal get less than those who exemplify
> the masculine ideal. Fewer resources are invested in the health and education of women;
> they have fewer economic opportunities, less political power, and less freedom of movement
> (Harari 2014).

Women are doing better now, but the question is raised as to whether "better" is
good enough (Gay 2014; Morgan 2019; Frances-White 2019). Some women have
indeed made it to the top, but according to Roxana Gay, this proves merely that

"some of us are lucky" (Gay 2014). Further up the ladder, women disappear (Lerer and Avgar 2018). This statement is supported by a 2016 report showing that by the time her first child turns 12, a woman earns, on average, a third less per hour than a man. This state of affairs has been coined the "motherhood penalty" (Rose 2019). Girls grow up expecting to play the "mother" role (Williams 2017). Societal imperatives of gender—learned from birth—make girls believe that motherhood is a woman's duty. As Jacqueline Rose points out, "there is a set of clichés a woman is being encouraged—or rather instructed—to think" (Rose 2019). This is more than a simple cliché, though, since one of the most influential and prevailing sources of motherhood as a woman's duty is the Bible.

Chapter 3 explores women's reproductive duty in the Bible. It examines Bible stories that have affected women on reproductive issues in human societies in the past and present, asks why a commandment to reproduce was needed, explores how "barrenness" in the Bible was resolved, and what fertility—and infertility—still represent for women. "Be fertile and replenish the earth" (Genesis 1:28) is the very first commandment that appears in the Bible, prefiguring the Ten Commandments.[3] Thus, the Bible, in fact, provides the first written source in antiquity of the political status of the womb.[4] During the creation of a new, omnipotent God, the political writers of the Bible (or their leaders) determined that having more people around was better for the group. It is plausible, however, that replenishing the earth during biblical times was not an easy commandment to follow and, therefore, had to be strongly marketed. Infertility trouble and its significance for women—barrenness—appear again and again throughout the Bible. Moreover, the first commandment is so crucial that even the four biblical matriarchs are barren and conceive miraculously with God's help.

According to Stephen Greenblatt, biblical stories are influential in the present time as well (Greenblatt 2017). Indeed, biblical reproduction marketing has been so successful that more than two millennia later, biblical teachings about women and their roles persist. To be a woman with child remains—explicitly and implicitly—a social directive. Childless women are—supposed to be—miserable and pitied. In the second decade of the twenty-first century, a woman's reputation may still depend on her [in]fertility (Knott 2019). At the same time, however, women are struggling to escape motherhood. In May 2021, for example, an article entitled "How do you convince people to have babies?" appeared on the BBC website (Hegarty 2021). The writer is a modern population correspondent addressing demographic declines in China and the United States. Evidently, demographic whims and policies addressing the womb persist in modern times.

Chapter 4 addresses demography. It examines the womb as an instrument in demographic wars and asks whether and why women enroll in this scheme, either

---

[3] The ten commandments include instructions to worship only the one God, to honor one's parents, and to keep the Sabbath, as well as prohibitions against idolatry, blasphemy, murder, adultery, theft, dishonesty, and covetousness.

[4] The Bible is the source of the three monotheist religions and their cultures in the modern world. Previous written sources may exist, but they have remained mostly unknown in present-day culture.

willingly or unwillingly. The chapter gives a brief overview of the history of birth control and its discontents; it explores the intervention of the law in demographics and describes current trends and societal determinants of fertility. It concludes by addressing the status of women in demography planning. Modern demography is concerned with "numbering the people" and understanding population dynamics.[5] Presently, family planning emphasizes the right of the individual to determine family size (as well as the potential contribution of family planning to national and global population problems).[6] But is it really the individual who decides? As seen above, reproduction in the Bible was powerfully—and effectively—placed as a woman's duty.

Ever since, demography policies affecting women have been a worldwide reality. Chinese policies, for example, encouraged women to have children and then not to have them.[7] During the last decade, policy in China has changed, allowing couples to have up to two children and then up to three. China has been notoriously blunt about reproductive policies; but Stalin, Hitler, and Ceausescu introduced reproductive decrees as well. Today, some people believe that women's choices should be respected, even if they result in population decline. Others, however, including current political leaders, such as Russian President Putin, Turkish President Erdoğan, and Brazilian President Bolsonaro, see population growth as a national imperative and high fertility as "a female duty" (Turner 2019). Pope Francis has also declared that "opting not to have children is a 'selfish choice'" (Gibson 2015). In Israel, having children—more than one—is a social requirement. On both sides of the Israeli–Palestinian conflict, the womb is considered a war tool.

Demography is now influenced by birth control and family planning novel ideas concerning reproduction that could succeed and thrive, thanks to the development of the pill in the 1950s.

Chapter 5 examines the advent of the pill and its history. It explores the life of women in the 1950s and what contraception and birth control meant in those days. It reviews the story of the four heroes to whom we owe this development, explores the successes and difficulties of its marketing, and observes what is happening today in the area of contraception.

In the 1950s, women recognized that the pursuit of opportunity required independence, and achieving that independence meant avoiding or at least postponing motherhood (Eig 2014). In addition, women who married at 19 or 20 were done—or wished to be done—with babies by the time they were 30. Contraception and birth control were what many women wanted. But the Catholic Church firmly opposed contraception. Moreover, back in the nineteenth century, the 1873 Comstock Law, in the United States, prohibited the trade in "obscene literature" and "immoral articles," which included birth control devices and information on such devices (Lewis 2019).

---

[5] https://iussp.org/en/about/what-is-demography.

[6] Social and political aspects of birth control. https://www.britannica.com/science/birth-control/Social-and-political-aspects-of-birth-control.

[7] Social and political aspects of birth control. https://www.britannica.com/science/birth-control/Social-and-political-aspects-of-birth-control.

So far, the methods used were ineffective and dangerous.[8] Yet women were willing to risk serious side effects, arrest, and even death rather than remain pregnant.[9]

The key players in the development of the pill were two female activists, Margaret Sanger and Katharine McCormick, as well as a brilliant biologist, Gregory Pincus, and a devout Catholic gynecologist, John Rock.[10,11] To make the idea of contraception more palatable to public opinion, health providers, and politicians, Sanger presented the notion of "family planning."[12] For many women, the advent of the contraceptive pill was liberating, as it gave them highly effective control over their fertility. Thanks to the pill, women could postpone pregnancy, finish college, go to law school and medical school, apply for jobs, and take leading positions in government and the anti-war movement and in the fight for equal rights.[13] Moreover, the advent of the pill produced a contraceptive mentality that assumes that people plan their reproductive lives (Campo-Engelstein 2019). The pill is often viewed as a key milestone for women's rights and one of the greatest inventions of the twentieth century (Lewis 2019).[14] However, women's struggle in the abortion camp is a different story.

Chapter 6 explores elective termination of pregnancy. It looks at the incidence of abortions worldwide, examines the legality of the procedure and the situation of abortion in the United States (as an example of a country in which abortion is legal) and in Israel (where abortion is illegal). According to the Guttmacher Institute's executive summary in 2017, the vast majority of abortions are the result of unintended pregnancies.[15] However, out of 163 countries on earth, only eight have no legal conditions for abortion (mostly from the former Soviet Union, including Russia).[16] Either abortion is illegal, or, if it is legal, the country's abortion legislation includes restrictions; and the more restrictive the legal setting, the higher the percentage of least-safe abortions. According to recent estimates, 23,000 women die

---

[8] Women swallowed lye (caustic soda) and gunpowder, placed leeches inside their bodies, poked themselves with knitting needles, threw themselves downstairs, hammered their abdomen with brickbats, and swallowed potions.

[9] https://www.pbs.org/wgbh/americanexperience/features/pill-dr-john-rock-1890-1984/. Accessed 20.10.2020.

[10] https://news.bbc.co.uk/onthisday/hi/dates/stories/december/4/newsid_3228000/3228207/stm.

[11] https://www.pbs.org/wgbh/americanexperience/films/pill/ThePill Accessed 30.10.2020.

[12] https://www.britannica.com/biography/Margaret-Sanger.

[13] https://www.pbs.org/wgbh/americanexperience/features/pill-and-womens-liberation-movement/ Accessed 20.10.2020.

[14] https://www.pbs.org/wgbh/americanexperience/features/pill-dr-john-rock-1890-1984/ Accessed 20.10.2020.

[15] https://www.guttmacher.org/report/abortion-worldwide-2017-executive-summary. Accessed 25.4.2019.

[16] https://www.guttmacher.org/state-policy/explore/overview-abortion-laws. Accessed 25.4.2019.

of unsafe abortion each year and tens of thousands more experience significant health complications.[17,18,19]

The United States is counted among the countries in which abortion is legal. However, restrictions by state are permitted—and mounting. This is, perhaps, not surprising, since even in "landmark case" Roe v. Wade in 1973 that legalized abortion in the United States, a woman's choice to terminate a pregnancy was not considered an absolute right. According to the judges, states did have some "legitimate interests" in regulating or prohibiting abortions.[20] In Israel, abortion is illegal. But Israeli law permits abortion under certain conditions.[21] A woman who wishes to terminate a pregnancy must appeal to a committee (two physicians and a person representing "the public"). She must request authorization by "the state" to determine what happens to her own body. On the other hand, help for women to become pregnant in the first place has been welcomed, celebrated, and copiously funded.

Chapter 7 explores assisted reproduction. It provides a brief description of in vitro fertilization (IVF) from a medical perspective and examines some aspects of its history—the social, scientific, and political background in which it developed. It explores the present depiction and promotion of IVF, and finally, asks whether women are coerced into IVF.

Women experiencing infertility were the background in which IVF could develop. More than four decades have passed since the birth of Louise Brown, the first child born as a result of IVF in 1978 (Steptoe and Edwards 1978), and today, it is difficult to imagine the world without assisted reproductive technologies (ART). Despite much initial resistance by the medical community and by society, viewed as "a threat to the very fabric of civilization," (Henig 2004) IVF has now firmly established its place in the clinical management of infertility (Revel and Simonstein 2009). ARTs have affected both reproductive practices and our view of reproduction, in general (Holm 2009). The arrival of laboratory-produced embryos and pregnancies achieved by medical intervention has changed our perception of human reproduction—further challenging the role of women in their reproductive tasks.

The most frightening thing about IVF was the prospect of abnormal babies. These fears rapidly fell away after Louise Brown was born. She was normal (Henig 2004). However, between 1978 and 1982, there were just four successful births with IVF

---

[17] https://www.guttmacher.org/fact-sheet/induced-abortion-worldwide. Accessed 12.2.2019.

[18] Interactive map Center for reproductive rights. The World's Abortion Laws. https://reproductive rights.org/worldabortionlaws. Accessed 2.2.2019.

[19] Preventing unsafe abortion June 26, 2019 https://www.who.int/news-room/fact-sheets/detail/preventing-unsafe-abortion. Accessed 25.8.2019.

[20] https://www.landmarkcases.org/cases/roe-v-wade. Accessed 25.4.2019.

[21] If the pregnancy results from rape; if the woman is under 18 or over 45; if the fetus carries a genetic disease; if the pregnancy threatens the woman's life, and if the pregnancy is the result of adultery.

worldwide;[22,23] clear evidence of how challenging the IVF procedure was. Nevertheless, the documented history of IVF does not include failed treatments during those years, or how many women underwent the procedure unsuccessfully. IVF has, in fact, constituted experimentation on human subjects without the subjects' knowledge.[24] Four decades later, in a special issue of the Fertility and Sterility journal (celebrating the 40th anniversary of IVF), the editors explain that the low implantation rates in the early days were "problematically addressed with aggressive ovarian stimulation protocols, often uncontrolled…" (Niederberger and Pellicer 2018) The writers maintain that "improved protocols" have been developed over this time. Yet women also respond differently to the current synthetic hormonal stimulation compound.[25,26] It appears that after experimenting with millions of women over four decades, resulting in improved IVF protocols, each woman who starts IVF treatment still becomes a new experiment.

In 2018, it was reported that 8 million IVF babies had been born in the 40 years since the historic first in 1978. Yet according to the last CDC report in 2017 and 2018, the success rate of IVF in the United States remained at 24.2% and 24%, respectively,[27] similar to the success rate reported in 2003 (Henig 2004). Moreover, while more IVF babies were born in 2018 than in 2017 (an increase of 0.2%), the number of IVF cycles increased by 7.6%.[28] Nevertheless, IVF may be one of the first rather than the last steps of fertility treatment.

In the twenty-first century, IVF seems to have a "Teflon reputation," as notwithstanding the low success rate and its perils, women subject themselves massively to the procedure.[29] Clinicians–investigators have a tendency to over-accentuate the positive (Elizur et al. 2006; Remennick 2009). Moreover, IVF may be a salvation for some women, but may mean imprisonment for others; as in the era of ARTs, optional childlessness in paternalistic societies (mainly but not only) has become unthinkable. Women who would like to have a child but are unable to conceive are likely to be met with the expectation that they should engage in IVF treatment (Holm 2009). Some authors claim the need to eradicate the coercive elements in pro-natalist ideology, not access to ART (Petersen 2004). But how such eradication should be achieved remains unclear (Holm 2009; Wright et al. 2004; Callahan and Simonstein 2009).

---

[22] Howard and Georgeanna Jones. https://www.pbs.org/wgbh/americanexperience/features/babies-bio-joness/ Accessed 2.3.2020.

[23] https://ivf-worldwide.com/ivf-history.html Accessed 3.8.2020.

[24] Leslie Brown, for example, realized that she was the first woman to become pregnant through IVF only when reporters started to chase her.

[25] https://ivf-worldwide.com/ivf-history.html Accessed 3.8.2020.

[26] For instance, in Israel, hospitalizations following IVF treatment are considered as "pregnancy complications" and not necessarily due to the IVF procedure.

[27] https://www.cdc.gov/art/artdata/index.html. Accessed 3.8.2020.

[28] https://monashivf.com/fertility-treatments/fertility-treatments/the-ivf-process/ Accessed 3.5.2019.

[29] https://monashivf.com/fertility-treatments/fertility-treatments/the-ivf-process/ Accessed 3.5.2019.

Chapter 8 presents the use—and misuse—of IVF in Israel, a developed country with a pro-natalist society. It focuses on the open-ended Israeli policy on IVF, admired by many (and regarded as the "North Star" for IVF policy), and presents a study on the effectiveness of this policy (Simonstein et al. 2014). This chapter concludes by asking whether IVF remains an ongoing experiment.

Israel's National Health Insurance (NHI) covers unlimited cycles of IVF for all Israeli women for up to two children in a given relationship, even if the woman has living children already. This policy claims to support a "woman's need" to have babies. However, is this permissive IVF policy successful? To answer this question, we carried out an empirical research in Israeli IVF clinics.

Some writers claim that the Israeli policy constitutes 100% of "IVF *optimal* utilization" (Nachtigall 2006). This notwithstanding, the question remains as to whether unlimited cycles of IVF are really "optimal" and if so, for whom. In Israel, the percentage of IVF births in 2017 increased by 10% since 2010; yet the number of IVF cycles during this time increased by almost 37%.[30] Thus, the higher rate of live births is due to the increased number of cycles per woman, (Simonstein and Mashiach-Eizenberg 2012) showing a similar pattern to the trend in the United States. Moreover, the average success rate of IVF (rated by live births) in Israel has remained constant for the last two decades at 16–17% of live births per IVF.[31,32] However the "cumulative" live birth rates with IVF, worldwide, are presented as very high, (Pelinck et al. 2008; Malizia et al. 2009) overall, the rate of success after seven *failed* attempts is zero or almost zero.

This raises the question of how many babies are actually born in Israel, with its limitless policy, after many unsuccessful cycles. To answer this question, we performed a retrospective analysis from a sample of women who began IVF treatment in 2000 and women who were in IVF treatment in 2010 in two IVF clinics, in central and northern Israel.[33] The research included 573 files reviewed during 2011–2013. The findings of this study confirmed the ineffectiveness of the Israeli open-ended policy (Simonstein et al. 2014).

It appears, nevertheless, that in the not-too-distant future, all women, and not only women experiencing infertility, may find themselves facing further reproductive risks and experimentation with the development of reprogenetics (Silver 1998).

Chapter 9 focuses on reprogenetics. Lee Silver coined this notion as he foresaw the merging of molecular genetics (i.e., gene editing) and assisted reproduction (i.e., IVF). This chapter explores healthcare allocation related to gene editing and the possibility of enhancing future generations, examining the crucial involvement of women in a scenario of enhancing reproduction. Reprogenetics with gene editing[34]

---

[30] In vitro fertilization (IVF) treatments 1990–2017. Report October 2019.https://www.health.gov.il/PublicationsFiles/IVF1990-2017.pdf. Accessed 27.7.2020.

[31] In vitro fertilization (IVF) treatments 1990–2017. Report October 2019.https://www.health.gov.il/PublicationsFiles/IVF1990-2017.pdf. Accessed 27.7.2020.

[32] https://www.health.gov.il/Subjects/Med_Inst/IVF/Pages/IVF-list.aspx. Accessed 5.8.2020.

[33] These clinics were chosen because of the multicultural background of the surrounding population.

[34] With CrispR/Cas, or any other enzymatic tool if proved safe.

could be used to solve issues related to healthcare allocation as humans now live long enough to become stricken with late-onset chronic diseases (The EU Summit on Chronic Diseases 2014; WHO 2015). The potential improvement to people's health may result, by and large, in substantial betterment to public health (Bostrom and Savulescu 2013). Enhancing future generations, however, will require IVF, which evidently requires the involvement of women in the process. Remarkably, women's necessary involvement in an enhancing scenario has not been discussed by its proponents (Bostrom and Savulescu 2013; Harris 2009; Savulescu 2006; Savulescu et al. 2015). This may well be because reproductive risks have always been part of a woman's life. But would it be fair to add the pain and risks involved in IVF to women's already challenging reproductive tasks?

The selection of healthy embryos for implantation with PGD already exists and involves women reproducing by IVF, albeit a relatively small group. Although enhancing future generations by editing the germline would require that *all* women reproduce using IVF,[35] the discussion about enhancing the germline, thus far, has focused only on future generations. Opponents of enhancement claim that modifying human embryos is dangerous and unnatural and does not take into account the consent of future generations. Proponents of enhancement focus on creating "better" offspring, disease-free and resistant to other maladies, and fitter overall (Harris 2005, 2007). Julian Savulescu also introduced the principle of procreative beneficence (PPB), stating that parents have the moral obligation to enhance their children genetically (Savulescu 2001).

The present discourse on moral obligations toward future generations does not refer to women but implies that all women pursuing motherhood may be required morally, if not legally, to reproduce with IVF (Simonstein 2006). According to Christine Overall, in an enhancing scenario, all women would be engaging in "a massive and dangerous medical experiment that includes bodily invasion, time, low success rate, and the risks related to a pregnancy with IVF" (Overall 2012). In my view, the implementation of the PPB would monstrously expand the already existing largest medical experiment on human beings: assisted reproduction with IVF.

Proponents of the PPB do not suggest allowing a government or social agencies to police pregnant women's behavior or make the PPB compulsory. However, as the title of this book reminds us, private decisions about reproduction have always been shaped by public laws and policies (Overall 2012; Solinger 2005).[36] Would women have the choice of whether or not to participate in an enhancing scenario? Would it become an obligation? Would it be a moral duty and/or a legally binding scheme? Nowadays, there is an ongoing discussion on "women's well-being" and "freedom" in reproductive matters. From this perspective, it is impossible to overlook Shulamith

---

[35] A vivid example of such a scenario can be seen in the 1997 film GATTACA. But the film does not focus on the necessity of all women to reproduce only through IVF. The film's focus is—as usual—only on the potential effects of enhancing regarding "optimal"—and sub-optimal—future generations.

[36] According to Solinger, this might be a difficult insight to bring into focus because of the way the idea of "personal choice" has obscured all other ways of thinking about pregnancy and motherhood (Solinger 2005) .

Firestone's work in the 1970s. She wrote that technology, i.e., artificial wombs (AWs), can liberate women from their biology and extend their choices (Firestone 2003). In a scenario of genetic enhancing, would ensuring women's autonomy and choice require the advent of the artificial womb?

Chapter 10 focuses on ectogenesis.[37] It presents the scientific and technological research indicating that the advent of the AW may be closer than we think. It focuses on the health and social tolls that reproduction takes on women, which could be avoided through ectogenesis, and discusses conundrums that ectogenesis may entail. The latest development on both sides of gestation, at its end (ectogestation) (Kleeman 2020)[38] and at its beginning (ectogenesis), (Rozenblum 2019; Kuperman et al. 2020), demonstrates that serious improvements have been made in the research on AWs. Ectogenesis might be a solution to avoid the need for a surrogate, for women who want a biological baby but lack a womb (for any reason), and for homosexual male couples. It might also, perhaps, appeal to women who may need IVF to reproduce.[39] Most importantly, it may prevent damage to women's health. The research on ectogenesis, however, is driven by the desire to save the lives of extremely low birth weight (ELBW) infants, by the requirement to improve embryo implant in IVF, and for growing tissue in laboratories for organ transplants (Lemme et al. 2018; Lee et al. 2018). Absent from the aims of the AW research is the improvement of women's health.

Why is this so? Some authors explain that maternity "is an essential function that women fulfill for the survival of our species" and that "reproductive hazards have traditionally been viewed as women's fate and taken for granted." However, the same authors add that a pregnancy may compromise women's health and can sometimes be deadly (Cook et al. 2003). Indeed, according to the WHO, in 2017, about 300,000 women died during and following pregnancy and childbirth.[40] And however most deaths due to reproductive labor occur in developing countries, about 700 women die each year in the United States as a result of pregnancy or delivery complications.[41] Even without a death sentence, for too many women, pregnancy itself still entails bad health. According to the CDC, pregnancy symptoms and complications can range from "mild and annoying discomforts" to "severe, sometimes life-threatening, illnesses."[42] The risks of a natural pregnancy include high blood pressure, gestational diabetes, severe, persistent nausea and vomiting, anemia, and preeclampsia (a serious

---

[37] Although ectogenesis and the artificial womb are not the same (ectogenesis is the process and the artificial womb is the tool), in this book I use these expressions interchangeably.

[38] http://www.w-cpc.org/news/reuter7-97.html. Accessed 13.7.2004.

[39] Women may save time, pain, bad moods, and endless frustration.

[40] https://www.who.int/news-room/fact-sheets/detail/maternal-mortality. Accessed 8.3.2021.

[41] https://www.cdc.gov/reproductivehealth/maternalinfanthealth/pregnancy-relatedmortality.htm. Accessed 8.3.2021.

[42] https://www.cdc.gov/reproductivehealth/maternalinfanthealth/pregnancy-complications.html. 20.8.2020.

condition that can lead to preterm delivery and death) (Lee et al. 2018).[43,44] IVF carries even higher risk (Skalkidou et al. 2017; Martin and Welch 1998; Pandian et al. 2005). Nevertheless, women are not supposed to complain.[45] We ignore the blood, the pain, and the stitches because that is the way things are. Indeed, most women had never questioned their reproductive role.[46] So far, the only way to avoid pregnancy discomfort, labor pain, and birth trauma had been abstention from pregnancy and childbirth (Kendal 2015). For some women, the option to have a genuine choice of whether (or not) to bear a child in order to become a parent could be of value.

Ectogenesis is not exactly welcomed, however, with most countries banning research on human embryos beyond day 14 (Final Report of the Royal Commission on New Reproductive Technologies 1993). In actual fact, the AW is highly controversial in academic discussion, (Singer and Wells 1984; Harris 1998) but little is known about the views of the general public in relation to these topics. Awareness of people's views on AWs could be useful for further discussion about ethical and legal conditions and for the development of adequate legislation.

Chapter 11 presents a pilot study of lay people's views on the advent of the artificial womb and ectogenesis (Simonstein and Mashiach Eizenberg 2009). The purpose of this study was to explore the attitudes of lay people in Israel—a pro-natalistic country that has eagerly adopted IVF—toward the advent of the AW. The study included 216 subjects aged over 21 who answered a structured self-report questionnaire examining the extent to which the respondent would use the AW in practice. The results of this study clearly suggest that further research on this topic is necessary.

References

Adrian, Leftwich. 2004. *What is Politics?* 428. Oxford: Polity Press.
Bostrom, N., and J. Savulescu. 2013 [2009]. Human Enhancement Ethics: The State of the Debate. In *Human Enhancement*, ed. Julian Savulescu, and Nick Bostrom, 1–24, 12. Oxford: Oxford University Press.
Callahan, D. 2009. Women, Work, and Children: Is There a Solution? In *Reprogen-Ethics and the Future of Gender*, ed. Frida Simonstein, 91–104. London: Springer.
Campo-Engelstein, Lisa. 2019. *Are We Ready for Men to Take the Pill?* Albany Medical College. https://www.bbc.co.uk/news/health-49879667. Accessed 20 November 2020.
Cook, R., B.M. Dickens, and M.F. Fathalla. 2003. *Reproductive Health and Human Rights.* NY: Oxford University Press.
Criado Perez, Caroline. 2019. *Invisible Women*. London: Penguin.
Dahl, Robert. 1957. *The Concept of Power*. https://fbaum.unc.edu/teaching/articles/Dahl_Power_1957.pdf. Accessed 3 June 2021.
Eig, Jonathan. 2014. *The Birth of the Pill*. London: Macmillan.

---

[43] https://www.nichd.nih.gov/health/topics/pregnancy/conditioninfo/complications.   Accessed 20.8.2020.

[44] https://www.mydr.com.au/babies-pregnancy/toxaemia-of-pregnancy. Accessed 1.8.2020.

[45] The first sin in the Bible, anyone?

[46] https://www.nichd.nih.gov/health/topics/pregnancy/conditioninfo/complications.   Accessed 20.8.2020.

Elizur, S.E., L. Lerner-Geva, J. Levron, A. Shulman, D. Bider, and J. Dor. 2006. Cumulative Live Birth Rate Following In Vitro Fertilization: Study of 5310 Cycles. *Gynecological Endocrinology* 22: 25–30.

Final Report of the Royal Commission on New Reproductive Technologies. 1993. Minister of Government Services, Canada. Ottawa: Canada Communications Group.

Firestone, S. 2003 [1970]. *The Dialectic of Sex*. NY: Farrar, Straus and Giroux.

Frances-White, Deborah. 2019. *The Guilty Feminist*. London: Virago.

Gay, R. 2014. *Bad Feminist*. London: Corsair.

Gibson, David. 2015. https://religionnews.com/2015/02/11/pope-francis-opting-not-children-sel fish-choice/. Accessed 20 October 2020.

Greenblatt, Stephen. 2017. *Adam and Eve. The Story that Created Us*. London: Penguin.

Harari, Y.N. 2014. *Sapiens. A Brief History of Human of Humankind*. London: Vintage.

Harris, J. 1998. *Clones, Genes and Immortality*. Oxford: Oxford University Press.

Harris, J. 2005. Scientific Research is a Moral Duty. *Journal of Medical Ethics* 31: 242–248.

Harris, J. 2007. *Enhancing Evolution: The Ethical Case for Making Better People*. Princeton: Princeton University Press.

Harris, J. 2013 [2009]. Enhancements Are a Moral Obligation. In *Human Enhancement*, ed. Julian Savulescu, and Nick Bostrom, 131–154. Oxford: Oxford University Press.

Hegarty, Stephanie. 2021. *How Do You Convince People to Have Babies?* https://www.bbc.com/news/world-57112631.amp. Accessed 21 May 2021.

Henig, M.R. 2004. *Pandora's Baby*. NY: Houghton Mifflin.

Holm, Soren. 2009. The Medicalisation of Reproduction—A 30 Years Perspective. In *Reprogen-Ethics and the Future of Gender*, ed. Frida Simonstein, 29–36. London: Springer.

Kendal, Evie. 2015. *Equal Opportunity and the Case for State Sponsored Ectogenesis*. Basingstoke: Palgrave Macmillan.

Kleeman, J. 2020. *'Parents Can Look at Their Foetus in Real Time': Are Artificial Wombs the Future?* 27 June. https://www.theguardian.com/lifeandstyle/2020/jun/27/parents-can-look-foetus-real-time-artificial-wombs-future. Accessed 20 January 2021.

Knott, Sarah. 2019. *Mother. An Unconventional Story*. London: Random House.

Kuperman, T., D. Elad, D. Grisaru et al. 2020. Tissue-Engineered Multi-cellular Models of the Uterine Wall. *Biomechanics and Modeling in Mechanobiology* 19: 1629–1639.

Lee, Jiyoon, Robert Böscke, Pei-Ciao Tang, Byron H. Hartman, Stefan Heller et al. 2018. Hair Follicle Development in Mouse Pluripotent Stem Cell-Derived Skin Organoids. *Cell Reports* 22 (1): 242. https://doi.org/10.1016/j.celrep.2017.12.007.

Lemme, Marta, Bärbel M. Ulmer, Marc D. Lemoine, Antonia T.L. Zech, Frederik Flenner et al. 2018. Atrial-Like Engineered Heart Tissue: An In Vitro Model of the Human Atrium. *Stem Cell Reports*. https://doi.org/10.1016/j.stemcr.2018.10.008.

Lerer, Michal, and Ido Avgar. 2018. *Representation of Women in the Israeli Academia*. The Knesset, Research and Information Center. https://m.knesset.gov.il/EN/activity/mmm/me040618.pdf. Accessed 22 April 2021.

Lewis, Jone Johnson. 2019. *The History of the Comstock Law*. https://www.thoughtco.com/history-of-the-comstock-law-3529472. Accessed 30 October 2020.

Malizia, B., M.R. Hacker, and A.S. Penzias. 2009. Cumulative Live-Birth Rates After In Vitro Fertilization. *New England Journal of Medicine* 360: 236–243.

Martin, P.M., and H.G. Welch. 1998. Probabilities for Singleton and Multiple Pregnancies After In Vitro Fertilization. *Fertility and Sterility* 70 (3): 478–481.

Morgan, Eleanor. 2019. *Hormonal. A Conversation About Women's Bodies, Mental Health and Why We Need to Be Heard*. London: Virago.

Nachtigall, R.D. 2006. International Disparities in Access to Infertility Services. *Fertility and Sterility* 85: 871–875 (53. IVF in Israel (in Hebrew) Ministry of Health). http://www.health.gov.il/Download/pages/IVF_1986-2009.pdf. Retrieved 28 June 2011.

Niederberger, C., and A. Pellicer. 2018. Introduction. *Forty Years of IVF Fertility and Sterility* 110 (2): 188–189. https://doi.org/10.1016/j.fertnstert.2018.06.005.

Overall, C. 2012. *Why Have Children? The Ethical Debate.* Cambridge: MIT Press.

Pandian, Z., A. Templeton, G. Serour, and S. Bhattacharya. 2005. Number of Embryos for Transfer After IVF and ICSI: A Cochrane Review. *Human Reproduction* 20 (10): 2681–2687.

Pelinck, M.J., H.M. Knol, N.E.A. Vogel, E.G.J.M. Arts, A.H.M. Simons et al. 2008. Cumulative Pregnancy Rates After Sequential Treatment with Modified Natural Cycle IVF Followed by IVF with Controlled Ovarian Stimulation. *Human Reproduction* 23: 1808–1814.

Petersen, T.S. 2004. A Woman's Choice?—On Women, Assisted Reproduction and Coercion. *Ethical Theory and Moral Practice* 7: 81–90.

Remennick, L. 2009. Childless in the Land of Imperative Motherhood: Stigma and Coping Among Infertile Israeli Women. *Sex Roles* 43: 821–841.

Revel, Ariel. 2009. Current Status of Assisted Reproductive Techniques (ART)—A 30 Years Retrospective. In *Reprogen-Ethics and the Future of Gender*, ed. Frida Simonstein, 15–28. London: Springer.

Rose, Jacqueline. 2019. *Mothers. An Essay of Love and Cruelty.* London: Faber & Faber.

Rozenblum, S. 2019. Making Life. 7 Days Supplement. *Yediyot Aharonot*, 12 April, 34, Hebrew.

Savulescu, J. 2001. *"Procreative Beneficience": Why We Should Select the Best Children.* Blackwell Publishing.

Savulescu, J. 2006. Genetic Interventions and the Ethics of Enhancement of Human Beings. In *The Oxford Handbook on Bioethics*, ed. Bonnie Steinbock, 516–535. Oxford: Oxford University Press.

Savulescu, J., J. Pugh, T. Douglas et al. 2015. The Moral Imperative to Continue Gene Editing Research on Human Embryos. *Protein and Cell* 6: 476–479.

Silver, M. Lee. 1998. *Remaking Eden.* London: Weidenfeld and Nicolson.

Simonstein, F. 2006. Artificial Reproduction Technologies (RTs)—All the Way to the Artificial Womb? *Medicine, Health Care and Philosophy* 9 (3): 359–365.

Simonstein, F., and M. Mashiach Eizenberg. 2009. The Artificial Womb: A Pilot Study Considering People's Views on the Artificial Womb and Ectogenesis in Israel. *Cambridge Quarterly of Healthcare Ethics* 18 (1): 87–94.

Simonstein, F., and M. Mashiach-Eizenberg. 2012. How Long Should Women Persevere with IVF? *Journal of Health Services Research & Policy* 17 (2): 121–123.

Simonstein, F., M. Mashiach-Eizenberg, A. Revel, and J.S. Younis. 2014. Assisted Reproduction Policies in Israel: A Retrospective Analysis of In Vitro Fertilization–Embryo Transfer. *Fertility and Sterility* 102 (5): 1301–1306.

Singer, P., and D. Wells. 1984 [1998]. *The Reproduction Revolution: New Ways to Making Babies.* Oxford: Oxford University Press.

Skalkidou, A., T.N. Sergentanis, S.P. Gialamas et al. 2017. Risk of Endometrial Cancer in Women Treated with Ovary-Stimulating Drugs for Subfertility. *Cochrane Database of Systematic Reviews* 3 (3): CD010931. https://doi.org/10.1002/14651858.CD010931.pub2.

Solinger, R. 2005. *Pregnancy and Power.* NY: New York University Press.

Steptoe P.C., and R.G. Edwards. 1978. Birth After the Reimplantation of a Human Embryo. *Lancet* 2 (8085): 366.

Turner, Adair. 2019. *Two Cheers for a Declining Population.* https://www.fnlondon.com/amp/art icles/two-cheers-for-a-declining-population-20190130. Accessed 3 June 2021.

Williams, Joanna. 2017. *Women vs. Feminism.* London, UK: Emerald Publishing.

Wright, V.C., J. Chang, G. Jeng, M. Chen, and M. Macaluso. 2007. Assisted Reproductive Technology Surveillance—United States, 2004. *MMWR Surveillance Summaries* 56 (6): 1–22.

Chapter 2
Man and Woman He Created

Do you remember when you first had a real sense of being male or female? How did this happen and what did it seem to mean? (Chakrabarti 2019, p. 19)

According to Shami Chakrabarti (2019), a person's sex identity is probably the first thing you notice and the last thing you forget about them. Crayson Perry (2017), in The Descent of Man, focusing on the identity of men, points out that one of the problems when talking about masculinity is the confusion between sex (male) and gender (man). Perry: "The physical, definite, pretty much unchanging fact of the male body can make us think that all the behaviours, feelings and culture associated with that body (masculinity) are also immutably writ in flesh." Perry observes that for many males, being masculine, acting in a manly way, is as "unquestionably a biological part of them as their testicles and penis and deep voice." But, he adds, "Masculinity is mainly a set of habits, traditions and beliefs historically associated with being a man." ...[and]... "a deeply woven component of the male psyche." (Perry 2017, pp. 4, 5).

We may doubt Crayson Perry's ideas and complaints about masculinity, since he is an outspoken transvestite.[1] But Lewis Howes, a former football player and the author of The Mask of Masculinity, also complains about the "traditional notions of masculinity," i.e., men "must work hard," "be tough," "win at all cost," "be aggressive," "be unemotional," etc. to which he subscribed for many years (Howes 2017, p. 1). Similar to Perry's claim about masculinity, femininity is also a "deeply woven component" of the female psyche. We may change the words "male," "man," "masculinity," "testicles" and "penis" that define male with the notions and organs that define female, woman, and femininity. If we change the words used by Perry, in the source, to define masculinity to words that define femininity, it goes like this: One of the problems when talking about *femininity* is the confusion between sex (*female*) and gender (*woman*).

---

[1] Here, I use the term that Perry uses to describe himself: "Maybe my circumstances, being a transvestite..." (Grayson (2017 [2016], p. 7).

© The Author(s), under exclusive license to Springer Nature Switzerland AG 2022
F. Simonstein, *Womb Politics: A Short History of the Future of Human Reproduction*,
The International Library of Bioethics 99,
https://doi.org/10.1007/978-3-031-11654-4_1

The physical, definite, pretty much unchanging fact of the *female* body can make us think that all the behaviours, feelings and culture associated with that body (*femininity*) are also immutably writ in flesh. For many *females*, being *feminine*, acting in a *womanly* way, is as unquestionably a biological part of them as their *ovaries and pubis and womb*. But *femininity* is mainly a set of habits, traditions and beliefs historically associated with being a *woman* [My version and my italics]. (Perry 2017, p. 4).

Chakrabarti observes, for example, that "wittingly or unwittingly," we teach boys and girls "to fit in" and know their "preordained place." So much so, she notes, that pink or blue products for babies, toddlers, and even older children might as well be "a neon-lit conveyor belt to our segregated prisons." (Chakrabarti 2019, p. 19). Chakrabarti grew up in the 1970s and experienced childhood in a decade, as she describes, "of apparent social progress in the UK, including in the relations between women and men." Nevertheless, she reveals that, on special occasions, she was dressed in "classic cartoon-like frilled dresses," was assigned "pink birthday cakes," and was bought dolls. Watching the boys around her highlighted the difference: "their clothes and birthday cake were blue and their toys were cars, swords and guns." (Chakrabarti 2019, p. 18). Furthermore, Chakrabarti exposes other "overwhelming" cultural influences on small children, from both inside and outside the home, which remain until today. Her own son, she writes, "seemed to be aware of the social significance of pink before he could even name the colour." (Chakrabarti 2019, p. 15). She corroborates Crayson Perry's address on the same matter:

> Masculinity and femininity are not primarily biological; they are mainly lifelong social routines we are schooled in from birth... By the time we are adults, most of us are consummate performers, passing as men or women effortlessly. (Perry 2017, p. 45)

This chapter examines notions of gender and its biases. It explores patriarchy and the theories that might explain its development in all human societies. In addition, this chapter examines the advent of feminism and looks at its discontents. Finally, this chapter explores motherhood and the notions of "womanhood" that may still be holding women back.

2.1 Gender

In 1955, John Money was the first to draw a distinction between biological sex, or the attributes that distinguish male and female, and gender—the behavior and roles that a person experiences and expresses. The word "gender" became popularized in the 1970s when feminists began to debate the rigid categories of social roles for men and women (Williams 2017).

Gender as a social construct has come to dominate thinking. It is assumed that society socializes people into thinking and behaving in a particular way according to the sex they are assigned at birth. Parents, friends and teachers think that some gendered lifestyle choices are appropriate for children, while others are not (Williams

2017). Chakrabarti writes, for example, that for her, sex and gender distinction became more and more real at school. "The physical space of the playground was seemingly eternally dominated by that permanent game of football engaging most of the boys while the girls were consigned to the margins to chat, skip or play games of imaginative role play." (Chakrabarti 2019, p. 16). Indeed, babies are born into an already existing world that comes with ready-made attitudes and assumptions about gender (Williams 2017). Perry, for example, notes that before they can spell their own names, children are well versed in the potent clichés of gender ; "girls play fairy dolls, make-up and gossip and a boy's world is full of space-ships, action and competition." (Perry 2017, p. 5). Nevertheless, the cultural expression of gender has changed over time. The history of pink, for example, shows that the symbols of masculinity and femininity can be totally arbitrary. We now see that pink is for girls; however, not many people know that, until the nineteenth century, pink was considered more suitable for boys and blue was for girls (Perry 2017).

At the beginning of the twentieth century, Simone de Beauvoir already referred to the arbitrary expression of gender when she wrote "one is not born, one becomes a woman." According to de Beauvoir, if you "become" a woman, then what it means to be a woman is negotiable. And if so, "under the right political conditions, you can un-become her too, you can shed the requisite role and make yourself" (de Beavoir 2019, p. 133). For the first half of the twentieth century, de Beauvoir's thought was revolutionary. Since then, many things have changed positively for women. However, are women now allowed "to make" themselves, in the third decade of the twenty-first century, as de Beauvoir suggested? Chakrabarti observes that the gendering of childhood in the last five decades "seems to have changed relatively little" and the stereotyping of toys and clothes may have now become even worse (Chakrabarti 2019, p. 16).

Gender Bias

> *Gender is a race in which some of the runners compete only for the bronze medal.*
> (Yuval Noah Harari 2014, p. 171)

> *Intellectual freedom depends upon material things...And women have always been poor, not for two hundred years merely, but from the beginning of time. Women have had less intellectual freedom than the sons of Athenian slaves.* (Virginia Wolf 2000, p. 106)

Criado Perez (2019) observes that most of recorded human history is one big data gap. Starting with the theory of man the hunter, the chronicles of the past have left little space for women's role in the evolution of humanity, whether cultural or biological. Instead, she notes, the lives of men have been taken to represent those of humans overall. "When it comes to the lives of the other half of humanity, there is nothing but silence" (Criado Perez 2019, p. xi). In the book Gender in History, Merry Wiesner-Hanks points out that even when the silence is broken, much of the record about gender, "is the story of women's subordination, which, it may make us, the readers, feel angry, depressed, or defensive." (Wiesner-Hanks 2001, p. 18). Throughout Wiesner-Hanks's research on women in history, she finds women playing a difficult role.

The historian and philosopher Yuval Noah Harari notes that, at least since the agricultural revolution, most human societies have been patriarchal societies that valued men more highly than women. No matter how a society defined "man" or "woman," to be a man was always better. According to Harari, patriarchal societies educate men to think and act in masculine ways and women to think and act in feminine ways, punishing anyone who dares cross those boundaries. Yet those who conform are not rewarded equally:

> Qualities considered masculine are more valued than those considered feminine, and members of a society who personify the feminine ideal get less than those who exemplify the masculine ideal. Fewer resources are invested in the health and education of women; they have fewer economic opportunities, less political power, and less freedom of movement. (Harari 2014, p. 171)

Many examples of historical gender bias exist. Stephen Greenblatt in Adam and Eve, for example, tells the story of the poet John Milton who, back in the seventeenth century, having become blind, demanded that his young daughters read to him, often in languages that they did not know. He taught them how to recognize and sound out the Greek, Hebrew, and other characters, but did not bother to teach them how to understand what they were reading. To his visitors who remarked on the strangeness of his daughters reading in so many languages without understanding, Milton replied: "One tongue is enough for a woman." (Greenblatt 2017, p. 200).

This happened four centuries ago, but at the beginning of the last century, Virginia Wolf was still not allowed to enter the "Oxbridge" library because she was a woman. Wolf quotes a Professor "X" saying that "women are intellectually, morally and physically inferior to men" (Wolf 2000, p. 110). This was Aristotle's thinking back in 400 BCE Athens. Evidently, the idea lingered up to Wolf's time. Today, many things have changed. A woman is allowed to enter an academic library unaccompanied by a man. Nevertheless, at the end of the second decade of the twenty-first century, Kate Manne still writes as follows:

> Masculine coded perks and privileges include social positions of leadership, authority, influence, money, and other forms of power, as well as status, prestige, rank, and the markers thereof...[and]... there are less tangible facets of social "face," like pride, reputation or standing, and the relevant absences – the freedom from shame and lack of public humiliation, which are more or less universally desired but only some people feel entitled to (Manne 2019, p. 113).

Coded perks and privileges? What is Manne complaining about? Things have changed, haven't they? The answer is yes. Perhaps, then, Manne is unjustly unaware of the positive changes by which women live, now, in the twenty-first century. As a transvestite man, Grayson Perry believes he is positioned at both sides of the gendered dimensions and, therefore, has a better perspective on gender issues. Perry claims that what millennia of male power have done is to make a society where we all grow up accepting that a system grossly biased in favor of "Default Man" is natural, normal, and common sense. According to Perry, Default Man is white, middle class, heterosexual, usually middle aged and feels he is the reference point from which other values and cultures are judged:

He has forged a society very much in his own image, to the point where now much of the other groups think and feel the same. They take the attitudes of Default Man because they are the attitudes of our elders, our education, our government, our media. … It is difficult to tweeze out the Default Man effect on our culture, so ingrained is it after centuries of its rules. (Perry 2017, p. 17)

Also writing about gender bias, Morgan (2019) observes that even with diseases that affect men and women in similar numbers, women are disadvantaged in their treatment. For example, men are 25% more likely than women to survive a heart attack, because women having a heart attack often present "atypically" (i.e., atypical for a man having one). Morgan notes that even recognizing female pain comes under massive gender bias in medical research, as the male body is the medical default. A study published in The Official Journal of the Society for Academic Emergency Medicine notes that compared to men, women often wait 16 min longer to receive pain medication in emergency departments and are 13–25% less likely to be given opiate painkillers (Morgan 2019).

2.2 The Patriarchy

Some women being empowered do not prove the patriarchy is dead. It proves that some of us are lucky. (Roxane Gay 2014, p. 182)

While undoubtedly many things have changed for women since the last century, and for the better, gender bias remains. Perry observes, for example, that when he talks to "many men" about a world "without the gross bias of the patriarchy," he feels like he is describing to them "a world without gravity, so fundamental is gender bias to their vision of reality." Furthermore, he tells that when he asked what is great about being a man, a member of a men's group said, "freedom, the feeling I can just do what I want." (Perry 2017, p. 17).

In *Sapiens: A Brief History of Humankind*, Yuval Noam Harari asks whether there are biological explanations for the preference given to men over women (de Beavoir, cited in Rose 2019). According to Harari, some of the cultural, legal, and political disparities between men and women may reflect the obvious biological differences between the sexes. In his words: "Childbearing has always been women's job, because men don't have wombs." Yet around this "hard universal kernel," every society accumulated layer upon layer of cultural ideas and norms that have little to do with biology (Harari 2014, p. 163). Harari argues that societies associate a host of attributes with masculinity and femininity that, for the most part, lack a firm biological basis. However, even though the precise definition of "man" and "woman" varies between cultures, he wonders whether there is some universal biological reason why almost all cultures valued manhood over womanhood. Harari explains that there are plenty of theories, "but none of them convincing" (Harari 2014, p. 172). Nevertheless, Harari points to three main theories in an attempt to explain the development of patriarchy. The next section examines Harari's three main theories.

1. *Men are stronger*

This theory points to the fact that men are stronger than women, and have thus used their greater physical power to force women into submission. A more subtle version of this claim argues that men's strength allows them to monopolize work that demands hard manual labor, such as ploughing and harvesting. This gives them control of food production, which in turn translates into political control. However, Harari notes that there are problems with emphasizing muscle power, for women are generally more resistant to hunger, disease, and fatigue than men. In addition, many women can run faster and lift heavier weights than many men. Moreover, and most problematic for this theory, women have, throughout history, been excluded mainly from jobs that require little physical effort, such as priesthood, law, and politics, while engaging in hard manual labor in the fields, in crafts, and in the household. Even more importantly, Harari asserts, there is no direct relation between physical strength and social power among humans. For example, people in their sixties usually exercise power over people in their twenties, even though youngsters are much stronger than their elders (Harari 2014).

2. *Aggression*

Masculine dominance results not from strength but from aggression. Millions of years of evolution have made men far more violent than women. Men are more willing to engage in raw physical violence. This is why, throughout history, warfare has been a masculine prerogative. Recent studies of the hormonal and cognitive systems of men and women strengthen the assumption that men have more aggressive and violent tendencies, and therefore, on average, are better suited to be soldiers. Yet granted that common soldiers are all men, Harari asks whether it follows that those managing the war and enjoying its fruits must also be men. To Harari, this makes no sense: "it is like assuming that because the slaves cultivating cotton fields are black, plantation owners will be black as well." (Harari 2014, p. 174).

3. *Survival and reproduction strategies*

Through millions of years of evolution, men and women evolved different survival and reproduction strategies. Men competed against each other for the opportunity to impregnate fertile women, and an individual's chances of reproduction depended on his ability to outperform and defeat other men. As time went by, the masculine genes that made it to the next generation were those belonging to the most ambitious, aggressive, and competitive men. A woman, on the other hand, had no problem finding a man willing to impregnate her. Harari:

> However, if she wanted her children to provide her with grandchildren, she needed to carry them in her womb for nine arduous months, and then nurture them for years, during that time she had fewer opportunities to obtain food and required a lot of help. Thus, she needed a man. (Harari 2014, p. 176).

This means that, to ensure her own survival and the survival of her children, the woman had to agree to whatever conditions the man stipulated so that he would stick around and share some of the burden. According to this theory, as time went by, the feminine genes that made it to the next generation belonged to women who were "submissive caretakers." (Harari 2014, p. 176). Women who spent too much time fighting for power did not leave those powerful genes for future generations. The result of these different survival strategies is that men have been programmed to be ambitious and competitive, and to excel in politics and business, whereas women have tended to move out of the way and dedicate their lives to raising children (Harari 2014).

Harari argues that this approach has no empirical evidence either. Particularly problematic, in his view, is the assumption that women's dependence on external help made them dependent on men, necessarily, rather than on other women, and that male competitiveness made males socially dominant; for there are many species of animals, such as elephants and Bonobo chimpanzees, in which the dynamics between dependent females and competitive males results in a matriarchal society. Though Bonobo females are weaker than the males, the females often gang up to beat males who overstep their limit (Harari 2014).

Indeed, some scholars have asserted that human society was originally a matriarchy in which mothers were all powerful; or at least egalitarian. For example, Peter B. Ellis, in *The Druids*, asserts that women had equal status with men in Celtic society until the Romans and Christianity arrived in the British Isles (Ellis 2002).[2] However, the evidence is ambiguous. According to Merry Wiesner-Hanks, the key problem in discussing primitive matriarchy is the lack of written sources (Wiesner-Hanks 2001). Nevertheless, Harari asks, if matriarchy can exist among elephants and Bonobos, why can it not exist among humans? (Harari 2014).

While Harari thinks that there is no answer to this question, I believe there is one: Female Bonobos and elephants give birth to youngsters that are capable of either walking behind or clinging to the mother immediately after birth. By contrast, Homo sapiens newborns are practically fetuses, incapable of walking or of even clinging on to their mothers. Human babies become toddlers only after about a year (or two), but remain dependent on adult care for many years thereafter. Bipedal walking was a great evolutionary mechanism as it allowed Homo sapiens to venture further in the dangerous savannah—but it demanded a heavy toll from Homo sapiens females. For while the birth canal of the females narrowed to retain the fetus, the human brain became larger.[3] As a result, childbirth became hugely hazardous for women and, frequently, a death sentence. If a woman was lucky enough to survive childbirth, she had to nourish herself and her baby. Broken and/or weak after giving birth and with a fetus now in her arms, a woman needed a man to provide for her and her baby, as the theory goes. Why could another woman not be her provider? Probably because

---

[2] A compelling story told by Ellis (2002) is the "Law of the Innocents" from AD 697 that, among other things, forbade women to be warriors or military commanders. Ellis tells that the ruler Adonan was moved to propose the new law, after an appeal by his mother, Ronnat, when they were crossing a battlefield together and saw the terrible sight of a beheaded woman with her child still suckling at her breasts; "a stream of milk on one of its cheeks and a stream of blood on the other" (p. 108).

[3] Independently of bipedalism.

the women around her were in a similar situation, i.e., either pregnant, in labor, or after childbirth.[4]

Most women may have had no problem becoming impregnated, but women had trouble holding on to the man to provide for her and the baby. Harari's mention of grandchildren seems farfetched. I am sure they were thinking of no such thing; all they wanted was food and protection to survive the day. Available sex for the man in question seems to have been an appropriate solution. Thus, to hold the man to provide for her, the Homo sapiens female "abandoned" the breeding cycles of all other species. For Homo sapiens males, sex became available at any time. Humans are also unique as the only species in which the female embellishes herself to attract the male. While in other species, the males compete for the females, in humans, the females compete for the males, to keep them around.

Scholars see the development of patriarchy as a complicated process, involving everything that is considered a normal part of civilization: property ownership, agriculture, the bureaucratic state, writing, hereditary aristocracies, and the development of organized religion and philosophy (Wiesner-Hanks 2001). However, the development of constant available sex was a huge survival accomplishment for the human female and, therefore, for the whole species. Women's embellishments also developed as a survival skill not only to attract the male, but more importantly, to make him stay. If men were indispensable for women's survival, they were obviously given the upper hand. A definitive answer to why matriarchy cannot exist among humans remains unavailable, but this theory on the development of patriarchy does make sense. In any case, it is the best we have.

2.3 Patriarchy and Its Discontents: Feminism

Not long ago women could not inherit property because we were property. (Deborah Frances-White 2019, p. 134)

True, a handful of women have made it to the alpha position, such as Cleopatra of Egypt, Empress Wu Zetian in China (c.ad 700) and Elizabeth I in England, yet they are exceptions that prove the rule. Throughout Elizabeth's forty-five years of reign, all members of parliament were men, all officers in the royal navy and army were men, all judges and lawyers were men, all bishops and archbishops were men, all theologians and priests were men, all doctors and surgeons were men, all majors and sheriffs were men, all students and professors in all universities and colleges were men, all mayors and sheriffs were men, and almost all the writers, architects, poets, philosophers, painters, musicians and scientists were men. (Yuval Noah Harari 2014, p. 171)

---

[4] A similar scenario is apparent in Call the Midwife, a TV series based on the memoirs of Jennifer Worth, a midwife working in East London during the 1950s. Before contraceptives were available, women were either pregnant, in labor, or with a baby on hands in this area of London. Worth, Jennifer (2012). Call The Midwife: A True Story of the East end in the 1950s. London: Orion Publishing.

Patriarchy was first challenged with feminist revolutionary thought following human rights and egalitarian ideals during the nineteenth century. Basically, feminism is the movement forwarded by brave and talented women (and men who joined them) who thought that women are capable of doing whatever a man does and should have equal rights to men. Nonetheless, feminist thought had first to conquer women's own longstanding beliefs. A century ago, Virginia Wolf was lecturing women in this vein:

> Young women, ... you are, in my opinion disgracefully ignorant. You have never made a discovery of any sort of importance. You have never shaken an empire or led an army into battle. The plays of Shakespeare are not by you, and you have never introduced a barbarous race to the blessings of civilization. What is your excuse?... It is all very well for you to say, pointing to the streets and squares and forests of the globe swarming with black and white and coffee-coloured inhabitants, all busily engaged in traffic and enterprise and love making, we have had other work on our hands. Without our doing, those seas would be unsailed and those fertile land a desert. We have borne and bred and washed and taught, perhaps to the age of six or seven years, the one thousand six hundred and twenty-three million human beings who are according to statistics, at present in existence, and that, allowing that some had help, takes time. (Wolf 2000 [1928], p. 110)

Indeed, women have had a longstanding engagement with reproduction. According to a census in April 2019, the number of human beings was 7.7 billion. However, many things have changed for women since Wolf's time. In The End of Men, for instance, Hana Rosin expresses her view that women have now risen and are powerful while it is men who are left behind because they are less valued and, in many cases, jobless (Rosin 2013). Eleanor Morgan also writes that, today, women lead. Morgan:

> We have achieved glory and greatness in industry, politics, law, science, technology, space travel, art, music, sport and so much more in all corners of the world. We have changed the world. (Morgan 2019, p. 182)

But she immediately adds: "And yet." Morgan describes women's enormous achievements at the beginning of the twenty-first century, but at the same time has her reservations. Roxana Gay echoes Morgan's qualms when she writes:

> 'Better' is not good enough and it is a shame that anyone would be willing to settle for so little. (Gay 2014, p. 100)

As Deborah Frances-White (2019) also points out, many of the structures and attitudes of the patriarchal era remain, and we live with the residue.

It is not only men who may retain patriarchal attitudes, however. Women have been conditioned into patriarchal ideals of womanhood and femininity for so long that there are women who may be willing to perpetuate these ideals.[5]

Feminism and Its Discontents

Frances-White runs a show in which she and her guests "confess" about times "when women's actions and values have spent time apart." She refers to "feminist values"

---

[5] At the end of the day, it is women who tied the feet of girls in China to comply with some masculine fetishism about women; and it is women who hold the girls in the female circumcision practice.

(whatever they might be) against what she and the women she interviews "do in real life." Frances-White and her guests always start each episode with one-liners that begin, "I am a feminist *but*…" According to her, these "confessions" are "playful, silly things that do not really matter" (Frances-White 2019, p. 20). For example, women becoming "bridezillas" for their weddings.[6] Frances-White's show starts by criticizing feminist ideals, but ends up as a funny, witty, and entertaining kind of self-criticism (Frances-White 2019). Yet some women's critique of feminism is neither mild nor playful. Joanna Williams, for example, writes as follows:

> There is a dominant feminist narrative that fills newspaper columns, book shelves, speeches at the United Nations and guidance for teachers… this narrative espouses one idea above all others, that women are disadvantaged and oppressed; routine victims of everyday sexism, casual misogyny and the workings of patriarchy… the better women's lives become, the harder it seems that a new generation of feminists must try to justify their purpose through uncovering ever more obscure problems… If women are to continue to live as equals to men and play a full role in forging the world for future generations, they need to throw off the shackles of feminism… (Williams 2017, p. 261)

This is a serious attack against feminism, but it is not the first. In the 1970s, Shulamit Firestone (2003) complained that "the daughters of a wasted generation no longer even knew there had been a feminist movement." According to Firestone, the cultural backlash following first-wave feminism was to be expected:

> Men…grasped immediately the true nature of a feminist movement, recognising it as a serious threat to their open and unashamed power over woman. They may have been forced to buy off the women's movement with confusing surface reforms – a correction of the most blatant inequalities on the books, a few changes of dress, sex, style ("you've come a long way, baby"), all of which coincidently benefitted women. But the power stayed in their hands. (Firestone 2003, pp. 23–24)

Nevertheless, Williams (2017) has a point. Girls, unlike in most of human history, can now go to school (Radcliffe 2013).[7] Girls now do better at school than boys, with the biggest attainment gap in reading, writing, speaking, and listening (but boys do better in maths and science).[1] In England and Wales, by the time they are 16, girls perform significantly better than boys in national assessments. Similar patterns are seen in the US (Radcliffe 2013). Joanna Williams (2017) also observes

---

[6] While the marriage tradition itself is the Patriarchy Special with a side of People As Property, Frances-White notes that brides can be "notoriously peculiar, demanding and emotional about their 'big day.'" Big weddings, she writes, "are superficial, narcissistic and 'actual madness' and the opposite of feminism." However, Frances-White reaches the conclusion that some women become "bridezillas" because it might be the only time in their life that they are in complete control of everything in their domain and they can. This is a woman's day: Her day, her space, her dress, wholly hers. According to Frances-White, a woman takes control of this day not because she cares more about pink tea roses than political influence, but because roses is all that is on offer. "Wedding trappings might be a superficial distraction, but they are also, for some women at least, a temporary power grab at a threshold of life recapitulation." (Frances-White 2019, p. 299).

[7] A fascinating novel telling the story of a woman who, in the Middle Ages, disguised herself as a boy to attain schooling is Pope Joan, by Donna Woolfolk Cross. Cross, Woolfolk D. (2005 [1996]). NY: Ballantine. Tales about singular women disguising themselves as boys to be able to learn are found also in Jewish folklore.

that some British universities now have twice as many female undergraduates as males. According to the U.S. Department of Education, National Statistics 2015, in America, almost 60% of all bachelor's degrees are awarded to women. These data are similar to the most recent statistics of 2019, published in 2021.[2] In 2015, young British women were 35% more likely to go to university than their male peers and 57.5% of students were female. In 2015, U.S. universities awarded more PhDs to women, and this has been the case every year since then.[3] In 2015, American women taking postgraduate degrees outnumbered men by 135–100 (Williams 2017). The most recent statistics of 2019 in the US (published in 2021) are similar as well as recent reports in the UK.[4]

In Israel, too, the number of women studying for all academic degrees exceeds that of men. In 2016/7, in academic institutions in Israel, 59% were women—58% of BA students, 63% of MA students, and 53% of PhD students. The two fields of study at universities in which women are most represented are education and teacher training (79–83% of BA, MA, and PhD students) as well as paramedical subjects (81–85%). On the other hand, the fields of study with the lowest representation of women are physical sciences (36–38%); mathematics, statistics, and computer science (26–33%), and engineering and architecture (27–31%).[5] The report notes that the gender breakdown in the various fields of study is not unique to Israel, and the rate of female students in the various fields is generally similar between Israel and the other OECD countries (Lerer and Avgar 2018).

Accordingly, if women are doing so well, Williams's continued attack against feminism should not come as a surprise: "Feminism needs to let women off the hook…women's freedom to make choices about their lives is to be celebrated." She blames feminism for holding women back today. In her words: "Women now need to liberate from feminism." (Williams 2017, p. 90).

But is she right? Deborah Frances-White (2019) reminds us that our life these days:

> is the direct consequence of the hopes of long-dead women…we live their hopes every time we walk down the streets unchaperoned, uncorseted, uncensored… every time [we] decided if, when and how to have a child and each time women do not die in childbirth because of the medical advances that are now our normal. (Frances-White 2019, p. 319)

We are the living, breathing manifestations of the hopes of women who are not breathing anymore. Should we now "liberate from feminism," as Williams suggests? It is true that women are doing much better; but it is true also that they disappear further up the ladder. Women are now doing numerically better than men in higher academic degrees, including in Israel. But in the 2015/2016 academic year in Israel, the percentage of women among the highest-ranking faculty members— tenured professors—was a mere 17% at universities and 15% at colleges (Lerer and Avgar 2018).[6]

Figure 1.1 shows the percentage of women in full-time equivalent (FTE) senior faculty positions at Israeli universities, by rank, in the academic year 2015/16. While women make up more than half of the lecturers, their disappearance further up the

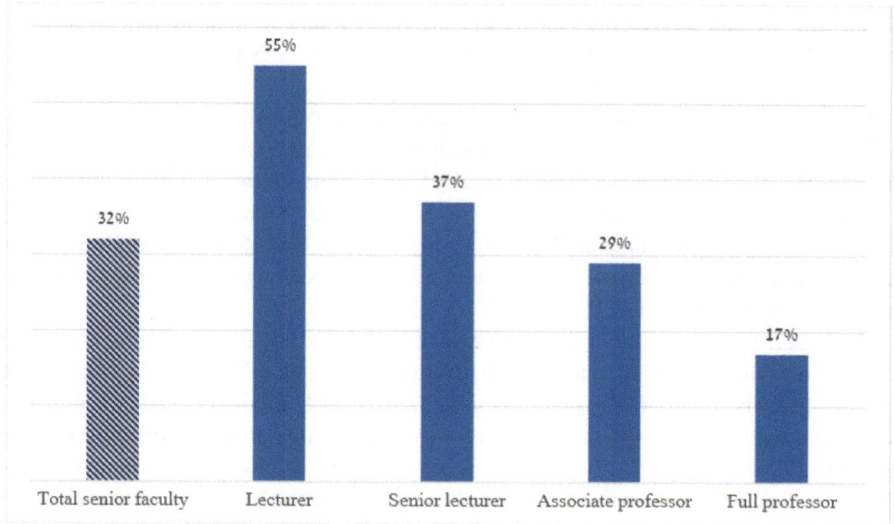

Fig. 1.1 Percentage of women in senior faculty positions (FTEs) at Israeli universities, by rank (2015/2016) (Lerer and Avgar 2018)

ladder, among the higher ranks of academia, is glaring. A similar pattern is observed in other countries (Lerer and Avgar 2018).

Williams herself conveys some confusion, as she notes that women are doing better than ever before, particularly when younger, and better than men "on paper." She explains also that the achievements of girls in the lower ranks "may indicate that they are better at *complying with the implicit and explicit rules* a new type of education involves" and that far more than boys, as "*girls are still socialised to conform and 'be good.'*" [my italics] (Williams 2017, p. 20). Williams:

> A ...price to be paid for school success may come later in life. Although girls' diligence and obedience is rewarded with certificates that help them secure a university place and enter well-paid professional careers, it may be less beneficial in the long term. Women are made into capable and diligent employees but progressing to the higher levels of some careers can require leadership, risk taking and an element of self-promotion. *These tend to be the very qualities girls have been socialised out of through their education* [my italics]. (Williams 2017, p. 27)

Is this not what feminists actually complain about? Moreover, could it be that women disappear further up the ladder not only because they "are made into capable and diligent 'employees,'" as Williams suggests, but also because women "are made" into capable, diligent—and mostly obedient—'mothers?'".

2.4 Motherhood

The education of girls formed no part of their vision. Their most fervent wish was for their daughters to get married...have children and settle down. (Jacqueline Rose 2019, p. 189)

It appears that parents still want to see their daughters settled down, married, and mothering children. Not surprisingly then, Judith Warner writes that in the "Mommy Mystique" atmosphere, "too many of us allow ourselves to be defined by mother-hood." (Cited in Williams 2017, p. 87). It is with this definition by women them-selves, carefully conditioned from early childhood (girls playing with baby dolls) that women get stuck on the way up the ladder, in academia and almost everywhere. On this matter, Hana Rosin (2013) writes that it was her own choice to work only four days a week after giving birth.

I also chose not to return to my studies until my second child was 6 years old. I thought that when he would reach the stage of elementary school—with so many new things to do and learn—my presence would be less necessary. It was my choice. But was it? I brought this child into the world and he needed me. I felt it was my responsibility to give him the best start. I do not know if I was right on this, but I waited dutifully. I started university only at the age of 29 and I was very lucky. Most women, after having children, cannot develop a career as I did.

Moreover, the subject of mothers is thick with idealizations, for instance, of the "perfect mother." Attachment parenting, for example, recommends that breast-feeding be more or less non-stop. Mothers are instructed to devote themselves wholly to their babies, step out of the career track, and according to some advice, "subju-gate yourself to your baby or else." (Rose 2019, p. 85). If this is the tone and the music, no wonder women who have succeeded in developing a career before having children disappear further up the ladder. Rose also asks why, in modern times, the participation of mothers in political and public life is seen as the exception:

> Why are mothers not seen as having everything to contribute, by dint of being mothers, to our understanding and ordering of public, political space? Instead, mothers are either being exhorted to return to their instincts and stay at home, or to make their stand in the boardroom – to "lean in"... – as if being the props of neo-liberalism were the most that mothers can aspire to, the highest form of social belonging and agency they can expect. (Rose 2019, p. 17)

The exclusion of women from the ladder altogether may begin even earlier, when a woman becomes pregnant; or even before, just by the thought that a young woman may become pregnant. In July 2015, a report issued by the Equality and Human Rights Commission stated that, every year, 54,000 women lose their jobs as a result of their pregnancy; double the number reported in 2005. Attention has recently focused on the gender pay gap that emerges when people have children—what has been labelled "the motherhood penalty."

A report in 2016 showed a gradual but continual rise in the average hourly pay gap, from virtually zero when men and women begin their working lives, to about 10% when a woman first gives birth. By the time her first child turns 12, women are earning, on average, a third less each hour than men (Rose 2019). Williams, however, argues that the gender pay gap "is not so much a motherhood penalty as a time away from paid work penalty" (Williams 2017). Reading this I wanted to laugh; and cry. For why is it that a woman has "time away from paid work?" Is it not because she has become a mother? Furthermore, Williams writes that women who "readily define themselves by motherhood" are more likely to feel guilty about working full-time and prioritizing their own needs: "they are more likely to leave work altogether for a few years or return part-time." (Williams 2017, p. 87). Some "poorly paid and tedious" work, she writes, can make staying at home a more attractive option, "especially for women that *grew up expecting to play this role.*" (Williams 2017, p. 71). She continues: "belief in a maternal instinct encourages them to begin preparing for their biological destiny." (Williams 2017, p. 77). Williams adds that she is in favor of a woman's choice, but she also points out that "choices are influenced by attitudes toward work as well as toward motherhood." (Williams 2017, p. 72). But if a woman has grown up "expecting to play a role," does this not mean that someone had inculcated this role in her mind? For as Jacqueline Rose also mentions, there is "a set of clichés" a woman "is being encouraged—or rather instructed—to think." (Rose 2019, p. 21).

Nevertheless, Joahna Williams continues to complain about feminists because "[they] are often quick to point out that the rhetoric of 'choice' is misleading and what may appear to be an individual woman's chosen life course is in fact the only option available to her." (Williams 2017, p. 72). In Williams's view, it is not "sexist bosses," "outdated laws," or "religious conventions" that prevent pregnant women playing a full part in society but "a view of women as nothing other than the carrier of a future baby." (Williams 2017, p. 81). Yet is this view of woman "as nothing other than the carrier of a future baby" not exactly what "sexist bosses," "outdated laws," and "religious conventions" are saying? Moreover, societal imperatives of gender— learned from birth, as observed above—make women believe that motherhood is a woman's duty (see also Chap. 2).

2.5 Conclusions

Whereas a person's sex—the attributes that distinguish males from females—is a biological determinant, gender—or the behavior and roles that a person experiences and expresses—are not. Gender is a social construct in which masculinity and femininity are a set of habits, traditions, and beliefs woven deeply as social behaviors in which we are schooled from birth by parents, friends, and teachers. We are taught that some gendered lifestyle choices are appropriated for us, while others are not. Thus, we become "women" and "men" by playing a predetermined role imposed by society. However, gendered roles have been biased and have favored men throughout human history. Theories explaining why patriarchal rules developed in all human societies remain unsatisfactory. Nevertheless, women's dependence on men because of the daily need for survival after giving birth has certainly played a role. The Feminist Movement that developed in the nineteenth century, following human rights and egalitarian ideals, started (at last) to demand rights and equality for women.

Women's lot has certainly improved, but disparities that favor men at the top remain.

While more girls than boys are doing better at school, college, and university, women disappear at the ladder, and those who make it to the top of their careers are the exceptions. What happens in the gap between the first steps of a successful woman's career and her advance up the ladder toward the top is having babies and raising children, getting stranded in the so-called "motherhood penalty."

In the context of womb politics, while motherhood is presently considered to be a woman's choice, after the advent of reliable contraceptives, is it really a choice? The most powerful gender imperative is that motherhood is not only women's capability—possessing a womb—but also a woman's duty. The next chapter examines one of the most influential and prevailing sources of this mandate in antiquity—the Bible.

Notes

(1) https://www.theguardian.com/education/2021/aug/13/girls-overtake-boys-in-a-level-and-gcse-maths-so-are-they-smarter. Updates. Accessed 15 Apr 2022.
(2) https://www.statista.com/statistics/236360/undergraduate-enrollment-in-us-by-gender/per centage in 2019. Accessed 1 May 2022.
(3) https://www.weforum.org/agenda/2018/10/chart-of-the-day-more-women-than-men-earned-phds-in-the-us-last-year. Accessed 1 May 2022.
(4) https://www.statista.com/statistics/236360/undergraduate-enrollment-in-us-by-gender/per centage in 2019. Accessed 1 May 2022; https://www.weforum.org/agenda/2018/10/chart-of-the-day-more-women-than-men-earned-phds-in-the-us-last-year/. Accessed 1 May 2022. https://www.theguardian.com/education/2021/aug/13/girls-overtake-boys-in-a-level-and-gcse-maths-so-are-they-smarter. Accessed 1 May 2022.
(5) The Israeli 2016/2017 statistics on gender in academia constitutes the most recent report to the Israeli Knesset. See Ferrero, Maria Anger (2020) The Culture of Genius and Women Impostors in Academia. Underrepresentation and discrimination of women in Academia. https://medium.com/the-faculty/women-under-representation-in-academia-3e950e02d699. Accessed 1 May 2022.
(6) This is the last existing report to the Israeli Knesset. See also Ferrero Maria Anger (2020) The Culture of Genius and Women Impostors in Academia. Underrepresentation and discrimination of women in Academia. https://medium.com/the-faculty/women-under-representation-in-academia-3e950e02d699. Accessed 1 May 2022.

References

Chakrabarti, Shami. 2019. *Of Women: In the 21st Century*. London: Penguin.
Criado Perez, Caroline. 2019. *Invisible Women*. London: Penguin.

de Beavoir, Simone, Cited in, Rose, Jacqueline. 2019. *Mothers. An Essay of Love and Cruelty.* London: Faber & Faber.

Ellis, P.B. 2002 [1994]. *A Brief History of the Druids.* London: Constable & Robinson.

Firestone, S. 2003 [1970]. *The Dialectics of Sex.* NY: Farrar, Straus and Giroux.

Frances-White, Deborah. 2019. *The Guilty Feminist.* London: Virago.

Gay, Roxana. 2014. *Bad Feminist.* London: Corsair.

Greenblatt, Stephen. 2017. *Adam and Eve. The Story that Created Us.* London: Penguin.

Harari, Y.N. 2014. *Sapiens. A Brief History of Human of Humankind.* London: Vintage.

Howes, Lewis. 2017. *The Mask of Masculinity.* London: Hay House.

Lerer, Michal, and Ido Avgar. 2018. *Representation of Women in the Israeli Academia (Hebrew).* The Knesset, Research and Information Center. https://fs.knesset.gov.il/globaldocs. Accessed 22 Apr 2021.

Manne, Kate. 2019. *Down Girl.* London: Penguin.

Morgan, Eleanor. (2019). *Hormonal. A Conversation about Women's Bodies, Mental Health and Why We Need To Be Heard.* London: Virago.

Perry, Crayson. 2017. *The Descent of Man.* London: Penguin.

Radcliffe, R. 2013. The Gender Gap at Universities. Where Are All the Men. *The Guardian,* January 29.

Rosin, Hana. 2013. *The End of Men.* London: Penguin.

Rose, Jacqueline. 2019. *Mothers. An Essay of Love and Cruelty.* London: Faber & Faber.

Wiesner-Hanks, Merry. 2001. *Gender in History.* London: Blackwell.

Williams, Joanna. 2017 *Women vs. Feminism.* London: Emerald Publishing.

Wolf, Virginia. 2000 [1928]. *A Room of One's Own.* UK: Penguin Classics.

Chapter 3
Womb Politics in the Bible

Humans cannot live without stories. We surround ourselves with them; we make them up in our sleep; we tell them to our children ; we pay to have them told to us...And a few of us – myself included – spend our entire adult lives trying to understand their beauty, power, and influence. (Stephen Greenblatt 2017, p. 2)

I came to have a heightened perception of the power the traditional story had over the sense of my standing in the world, especially when I travelled to places where the old social order was intact, where the small talk began with "are you married?" Or "do you have children?" (Emily Witt 2018, p. 203)

Emily Witt is single and in her thirties. In her book, The Future of Sex, she examines twenty-first century female sexuality. At some point, she wonders whether she would be happier if she could answer yes to the questions above: that she *is* married and *has* children. She enjoys her life. But she also knows that she would enjoy "the ease with which having a family could be explained, the universal approval with which it was met." (Witt 2018, p. 203). Indeed, in the twenty-first century as well, having a family is easy to explain and is met with "universal approval." It means, according to Witt, "settling down into convention."

Where does this "everyone's endorsement" (Witt 2018)—getting married and having children—come from? The biblical story of the first humans on earth, Adam and Eve, comes to mind. As Stephen Greenblatt notes, the Adam and Eve story has, over centuries, "decisively shaped conceptions of human origins and human destiny." (Greenblatt 2017, p. 3). This chapter examines the stories in the Bible that have affected women on reproductive issues in human societies in the past and present. It asks why a commandment to reproduce was needed, explores how "barrenness" in the Bible was resolved, and what fertility—and infertility—still represent for women.

F. Simonstein, *Womb Politics: A Short History of the Future of Human Reproduction*,
The International Library of Bioethics 99,
https://doi.org/10.1007/978-3-031-11654-4_2

3.1 Adam and Eve

Most scholars agree that the Torah as a whole, which is the first part of the Bible, was redacted more than two millennia ago, in the fifth century BCE (Greenblatt 2017). Nevertheless, according to Greenblatt, the story of Adam and Eve, which occupies only about a page and a half out of 1078 pages in the modern edition of the King James Bible, still works "brilliantly and effortlessly." Greenblatt:

> You hear it at five or six years old, and you never forget it... Something in the structure of this narrative sticks; it is almost literally unforgettable. In the long centuries since it was first told, it accumulated an enormous apparatus of support: teachers endlessly repeated it; institutions rewarded believers and punished sceptics; intellectuals teased out its nuances and offered competing interpretations of its puzzles; artists vividly represented it. (Greenblatt 2017, p. 6)

Greenblatt points out that few stories in the history of the world have proved "so durable, so widespread, and so insistently, hauntingly real." (Greenblatt 2017, p. 3). Moreover, while this is fiction "at its most fictional, a story that revels in the delights of 'make-believe,'" millions of people (including some of the subtlest and most brilliant minds that have ever existed), have accepted the Bible's narrative of Adam and Eve as the unvarnished truth. Notwithstanding the massive evidence accumulated by geology, palaeontology, anthropology, and evolutionary biology, Greenblatt notes that "untold numbers" of our contemporaries continue to take the tale as an historically accurate account of the origins of the universe and think of themselves as the literal descendants of the first humans in the Garden of Eden. Above all, ordinary people—who have listened to the story told from the pulpit, have seen it depicted on walls, or heard it from parents or friends—"grasped something crucially important about themselves." Somehow, the story of Adam and Eve speaks to all of us. Greenblatt: "It addresses who we are, where we came from, why we love and why we suffer." (Greenblatt 2017, p. 8). Moreover, although the story of Adam and Eve serves as one of the foundation stones of three great world faiths, it precedes, or claims to precede, any particular religion. Greenblatt claims also that whether we believe in the story or regard it as an absurd fiction, we have been made in its image:

> Over many centuries the story has shaped the way we think about crime and punishment, moral responsibility, death, pain, work, leisure, companionship, marriage, gender, curiosity, sexuality, and our shared humanness. (Greenblatt 2017, p. 39)

No wonder, then, that Emily Witt, and all women in the twenty-first century, are still expected to marry and have children. Other stories of human beginnings exist. Had history developed in a different direction, other ancient tales may well have served as our own bundle of origin stories and would undoubtedly have shaped us other than as we are. Yet the story told in the Bible persisted. If we accept Greenblatt's views on the influence of biblical stories nowadays as well, it is worth examining what the Bible writes about the womb.

3.2   The Womb in the Bible

Be fertile and replenish the earth. (Genesis 1: 28)

"Womb" is mentioned 56 times in the Old Testament and 71 times in the Bible overall. Out of 622,700 words in the Old Testament, 56 is not a great number. Nevertheless, the womb remains a key feature in biblical stories, which provide the first written source in antiquity of its political status.[1] Moreover, *"Be fertile and replenish the earth"* is the very first mandate that appears in the Bible; prefiguring the Ten Commandments.[2] This commandment is so important that it appears twice in the book of Genesis: the first time in the first chapter of Creation (Genesis 1: 28) and again in the story of Noah, after the flood in which God erases all the creatures he has created (Genesis 9: 1).[3] This commandment is somewhat puzzling, however, since conception is not unusual after a sexual encounter between a man and a woman. Why the need for a commandment to reproduce when it is such a commonplace occurrence? One explanation is that the Book of Genesis presents an etiological account of the world,[4] so the writers of the Bible were trying to explain how the world began.[5] Nevertheless, even if this explanation holds, the fact that "Be fertile and replenish the earth" is God's very first commandment to humans is still very odd. Someone had taken the trouble to write it down, above all other decrees, as an important *duty*.

In a society that has grown so large that people no longer know each other, duties, permissions, and prohibitions develop into laws.[(1)] Societies make rules and legislation to introduce some level of order (e.g., all cars must travel on the right side of the road) and to avoid free riding (e.g., taxes for all or mandatory army service). But the existence of a law that dictates certain behavior in itself indicates the need for such a law; implying that some parts of society were doing the opposite before the legislation was passed. The Ten Commandments introduced the precept of worshipping only one God because people were in the habit of worshipping many gods. We may assume that the commandments prohibiting killing and theft were included for the same reason: that people committed murder and robbery (as is still the case today). Despite the lack of direct evidence, it is plausible that the origin and purpose of biblical commandments either prohibited or encouraged actions that people did or did not do, respectively. This having been acknowledged, the next question to arise is why procreation is the very first commandment in the Bible. It is

---

[1] The Bible is the source of the three monotheistic religions and their cultures in the modern world. Previous written sources may exist, but remain mostly unknown in present culture.

[2] The Ten Commandments include instructions to worship only the one God, to honor one's parents, and to keep the Sabbath, as well as prohibitions against idolatry, blasphemy, murder, adultery, theft, dishonesty, and covetousness.

[3] Interestingly, agnostic women in Israel—and even believers—are unaware that *"Be fertile and replenish the earth"* is the very first mandate in the Bible. (This statement is not scientific; it is based on a personal survey.)

[4] I am grateful to Dr. Ada Geva for this explanation.

[5] Many such explanations exist; however, the explanation given in Genesis has survived and remains alive in the cultures originating in the three monotheist religions.

highly improbable that people abstained from sex, and conception after heterosexual encounters is not unusual. Since we can assume that pregnancies occurred naturally, in biblical times, and earlier, why then did reproduction have to be the subject of a commandment at all? Let us turn to some other stories in antiquity that may help to answer this question.

The Babylonian epic of creation, for example, tells the Mesopotamian creation myth, Enuma Elish: in the beginning, the stream of fresh water—the god Apsu—ran into the salty sea water, the goddess Tiamat. From this primordial intercourse, all the other gods in the Babylonian pantheon were born (Greenblatt 2017). But far from celebrating reproduction as an unambiguous blessing, the story focuses on a parent's potential for murderous rage when its quiet is disturbed. The newly created gods proved to be intolerably noisy, and the primordial father, Apsu, unable to rest, eventually decided to destroy his offspring. If the ability to rest meant killing the children, then so be it. But one of his sons killed him first. Now the primordial mother, Tiamat, sought revenge for the murder of Apsus, and waged war on her offspring to kill them. But she too was killed, by her grandson (Greenblatt 2017). In the Babylonian epic, "motherly instinct" and "good parenthood" ideals were, evidently, as yet unknown.

Besides being terribly noisy, as described in the Mesopotamian myth, childcare was always difficult, throughout history until today. Could it be that, in pre-biblical times, babies born naturally following heterosexual intercourse were left behind? This is an awkward question by modern-day standards of motherhood and ideals of motherly feelings as a woman's inborn character, but it may actually explain the first commandment in the Bible.

There is no evidence of child abandonment in the Bible, but in a historical novel set in Middle Age England, two millennia later, Ken Follett depicts a heartbreaking scene of a newborn left at his mother's tomb (Follet 1989). The mother—like many women in the Middle Ages—had died immediately after giving birth. The father was left with two other children to care for, who—like other children at that time in Europe—had to survive on dry bread and beer. Feeling incapable of caring for a newborn baby, he abandoned him to die with his mother.[6] The characters in Follett's novel are fictional, but this kind of event is authentic to the Middle Ages. A newborn's chance of survival was slim if the mother had died, in the absence of another woman available to breastfeed the orphan. Follett's tale resonates with the fact that, for women, a pregnancy is dangerous. Follett focuses on the Middle Ages, rather than on antiquity, but Rachel, the fourth matriarch in the Bible, also died in childbirth.

Indeed, childbirth has always been—and remains—a dangerous process. Even during the second decade of the twenty-first century, about 350,000 women died in childbirth each year, mostly in developing countries.[(2)] In developed countries, medical care has greatly lowered the rate of women's mortality during or soon after childbirth. However, nursing babies and providing for toddlers remains challenging today, even without disease, malnutrition, or both. Could it be that in pre-biblical

---

[6] In Follett's story, the child survived because a monk passed by, heard the baby crying, and brought him to his monastery, where he was raised.

times, even if the mother survived childbirth, newborns—totally dependent as they are and remain so for many years to follow—were abandoned?

Again, this is a difficult question by present standards of childcare. Yet in the 1990s, while researching infant nutrition, a pediatrician in Brazil told me that poor Brazilian mothers would come to the hospital emergency room with a baby in their arms. While waiting in the ER, having not eaten for several days, the mother would usually faint, and would then be admitted to the hospital with her baby. After 24 h— during which both mother and baby had eaten four meals—she would be released from the hospital; until the next time (personal communication). Poor Brazilian mothers found a way to avoid starvation, by turning to a hospital emergency room. In pre-ancient times, a parturient woman could not know whether, where, and when she would eat again.[7] In this situation, the odds of survival for both mother and baby must have been low, and the woman improved her chances by abandoning the newborn. This could be the answer to God's first commandment. It is plausible that political philosophers in biblical times understood that a larger group could be stronger. During creation of a new, omnipotent God, reproduction became a primordial issue since the existence of more people—more children, in the first place—was better for the group.

3.3   Infertility

Being 'barren' is hard where childbearing is central to a person's reputation or when childlessness is involuntary. (Sarah Knott 2019, p. 32)

The first commandment of the Bible, to be fruitful and replenish the earth, is, in fact, the first evidence of political and demographic whims attached to the womb. It seems, however that, in biblical times, replenishing the earth was no easy commandment to follow and therefore had to be strongly marketed; infertility trouble and its significance for women—barrenness—appears throughout the Bible, over and over again.

According to present medical sources, *infertility* is defined as the inability to become pregnant despite having frequent, unprotected sex for at least a year.[(3)] However, the Hebrew word for infertility, *Akarut*, is translated into English in the Bible as "barrenness." In English, this word has a derogatory connotation, such as in the following dictionary definition: "Often Offensive. Not producing or incapable of producing offspring. Used of women".[(4)] Indeed, "barrenness" precisely addresses the status of infertile biblical women. The Bible tells us that barrenness is a woman's worst curse. It is a Divine curse, producing an extremely humiliating status for women, both at home and in society at large. Moreover, although women are the ones who bear children, the first commandment in the Bible is incumbent

---

[7] As noted in the previous chapter, in female humans, providing unlimited sex may have developed to keep the male around, to care for her and the newborn.

on men, but not on women. If the woman cannot conceive, though, she is the one to be blamed. Her womb has been cursed and this is the reason she remains barren, but because her womb is closed, her man cannot fulfill God's first commandment. In addition, the child born to a barren woman blessed by God to conceive, through a miracle, would become an important and/or a heroic person.[5] The teaching "to reproduce and replenish the earth" is so crucial that even the four Jewish matriarchs in the Bible, who were certainly important women, were barren.

The next section addresses the stories of barren women in the Bible.

Barren Women in the Bible

Sarah

Sarah is the first matriarch in the Jewish tradition, and she is barren. She is so upset that she gives her servant, Hagar, to Abraham, her husband, as a means to give him the child that she has not been able to bear for him. In this way, Abraham could fulfill God's command to "be fertile and replenish the earth." Hagar does conceive and delivers a firstborn son, Ishmail, to Abraham.[8] Sarah remains barren. One day, two angels visit Sarah to inform her that she will give birth to a son. Sarah laughs at them because she is too old to conceive. Against the odds, however, Sarah becomes pregnant and gives birth to a son. She names him Isaac ("laughter/he will laugh" in Hebrew), to remind her that she had laughed in disbelief when the angels brought her the news that she would bear a son in her old age. Isaac, her son, is the result of God's blessing and a miracle.[9]

Rebecca

Infertility trouble and miraculous conception return with the second matriarch, Rebecca. She is brought from Abraham's original land (Paddan Aram in Syria) to be Isaac's wife when he is 40 years old.[6] Since she is barren, Isaac pleads with God on her behalf and Rebecca subsequently conceives. According to the Bible, Isaac was "threescore" years old when Rebecca gave birth. This means that she had been barren for 20 years; until God intervened. When God assists barren women to conceive in the Bible, they are destined to give birth to important people. God speaks to Rebecca: "…Two nations are in thy womb, and two manner of people shall be separated from thy bowels…".[7] In the words of the anonymous narrator: "And when [Rebecca's] days to be delivered were fulfilled, behold, there were twins in her womb".[8] She gave birth to Esau and Jacob, who became the fathers of two separate nations.[10]

---

[8] Thus, the modern use of surrogate wombs and the scenes in the Handmaid's Tale already appear in the Bible.

[9] The rest of this story describes Sarah's jealousy and cruelty toward her servant Hagar and her son Ishmail. Sarah demands that Abraham send them away and Abraham dutifully obeys. God saves Hagar and Ishmail from death in the desert. In the end, Ishmail becomes the forefather of the Arab people. Isaac becomes the second forefather of the Jewish people, and Abraham is the first forefather in both traditions.

[10] Rebecca also deceived Isaac so that he would give his heritance and blessing to Jacob instead of Esau, the firstborn. See also Coopersmith, Dina. Women in the Bible. www.aish.com/jl/b/women/Women_in_the_Bible_Rivka.html.

Thus, according to the Bible in this story, God is fully in charge of Rebecca's womb; when she would conceive and whom her womb would engender.

Leah and Rachel
Leah and Rachel are sisters; both are married to Jacob, and both are barren. Leah is Jacob's first wife, and the third matriarch in the Bible. Jacob has worked for Rachel's father for 7 years in return for her hand in marriage. But Leah, Rachel's older sister, is given to Jacob instead. A week later, Jacob is allowed to marry his beloved Rachel, as well, having undertaken to work for another 7 years. The Bible tells us that Leah succeeded in conceiving at some point because God pitied her: "And when the Lord saw that Leah *was* hated, he opened her womb…".[9] However, the same verse continues: "but Rachel was barren." Consistent with the three Jewish matriarchs before her, Rachel is childless and is, therefore, miserable and envious of her sister: "Rachel envied her sister; and said unto Jacob, Give me children, or else I die. The anonymous writer notes two verses later: "And God remembered Rachel… and opened her womb".[9]

Samson's Mother and Hannah
Manoah's wife (who is nameless in the Bible) was the mother of Samson. She was barren until an angel arrived and told her that she would conceive a son who would liberate Israel from the Philistines:

> And the angel of the LORD appeared unto the woman, and said unto her, Behold now, thou [art] barren, and bearest not: but thou shalt conceive, and bear a son….and he shall begin to deliver Israel out of the hand of the Philistines.[10],[11]

Hannah, the mother of Samuel the Prophet, was barren also, until she prayed to God and pledged her child to lifelong divine service:

> [11] …O LORD of hosts, if thou wilt indeed look on the affliction of thine handmaid, and remember me, and not forget thine handmaid, but wilt give unto thine handmaid a man child, then I will give him unto the LORD all the days of his life, and there shall no razor come upon his head.[11]

Hannah conceived only after making her vow. She kept her promise. After weaning the child, Hannah brought him to Eli the priest, to serve God. The child grew up to become Samuel the Prophet, one of the most important figures in the Bible, with two books appearing under his name, Samuel I and Samuel II.

The common thread running through these stories is that since God's very first commandment is to be fruitful, the worst curse for a woman in the Bible is barrenness. God intervenes with women who suffer this curse by opening their wombs, resulting in the birth of important or courageous sons. The commandment is directed toward men, but even the four matriarchs in the Bible are barren and are able to conceive miraculously only following divine intervention. For women to be willing to reproduce, this is a marketing strategy at its best. The hopelessness of a childless

---

[11] Samson's mother's name does not appear in the Bible. Her son is important. She, the carrier of the future heroic figure, is not.

woman in the Bible is reiterated in Tamar's story, but she is childless for a different
reason.

Tamar

Tamar is the wife of Judah's eldest son. Judah is one of the 12 sons of Jacob, the
third patriarch of the Jewish people, and one of the founders of the 12 tribes of
Israel. Judah has three sons and takes Tamar to be the wife of the eldest, Er. As the
story goes, "Er was wicked in the sight of the LORD; and the LORD slew him."
So Judah instructs his second son, Onan, to marry Tamar so that her child will be
a descendant of his deceased brother. Onan marries Tamar, but does not like the
idea that the child will be his brother's heir rather than his own, and "spilled [his
seed] on the ground." The story continues that "this act displeased the LORD so he
slew him also".[12],[12] After the death of his second son, Judah is afraid to lose his
third son, Shelah, to this woman. According to the Bible, Tamar is not to be blamed
for the death of Judah's son. Nevertheless, Judah sends Tamar back to her father's
house, supposedly to wait for Shelah to grow up. However, Judah has no intention
of carrying this through. Tamar dutifully waits at her father's house, but as the years
go by, begins to understand that Judah will never give her the now adult Shelah. At
this point, she takes things into her own hands:

> Tamar hears that Judah will be travelling to Timnath, so she dresses as a harlot, covers herself,
> and waits at the side of the road. Judah does not recognize her. He asks for her "service," but
> has no money on hand to pay her; Tamar (the "harlot") asks him to give her his "signet," his
> bracelets, and his rings. Judah gives them to her. From this encounter Tamar conceives; and
> she dons her widow's robes again and returns to her father's house.[12]

Judah sends a servant to Timnath to retrieve his possessions, but the servant
cannot find the "harlot." Three months later, Judah hears that Tamar is pregnant. She
is brought to him to be burned because she has evidently whored; and widows who
have whored deserve death. But Tamar presents to the public the staff signet, the
bracelets, and the rings. Judah understands that he is the father and does not kill her.
He acknowledges that she is more righteous than him because he did not give her
Shelah as he had promised.[12] Tamar gives birth to twins, one of whom will be the
ancestor of King David.

What can we learn from this story? First, that a woman is a recipient of men's
"seed."[13] Second, that a widow must become the wife of her husband's brother for
continuity of her deceased husband's seed.[14] Third, spilling one's seed means a death
sentence.[15] Last but not least, although Tamar is not barren, she is still childless; and

---

[12] The verb "Le'onen" in Hebrew means to masturbate (after Onan). In Jewish Law, masturbation
is prohibited.

[13] This is very similar to the Greek concept of womanhood.

[14] This levirate law remains in modern Jewish Law. Nowadays, however, the brother of the deceased
can release his sister-in-law from the obligation to marry him by performing a ritual in which he
removes a shoe from his foot.

[15] No wonder, then, that up until the nineteenth century, homosexuals were sentenced to death, and
up until the last century, were sent to jail.

a childless woman is worth zero, nil, nothing. So much so, that Tamar has to dress as a harlot and steal her father-in-law's sperm. Moreover, she is almost killed for it, since a widow is allowed to become pregnant only by her husband's brother. But to be a childless woman is worse than death. Tamar had the resourcefulness to deceive Judah and survive. Moreover, her deceit and her trespass of the law went unpunished. Since conception and birth for a woman is a must, in her situation, according to the Bible, she did the right thing.

Most of the stories in the Bible about barren wombs—and the impossibility of this situation for women—have been passed down as they are to modern times. However, stories of barren women exist also in the Talmud.

3.4 Women in the Talmud

The Talmud is a compilation of oral legacy and interpretation of biblical passages, assembled over a period of 300 years, from the second century CE. The Talmud, its teachings (and teachers) were fiercely attacked during those times; nonetheless, the texts have survived intact until today. Nowadays, the Talmud is the central text of Rabbinic Judaism and the primary source of Jewish religious law and Jewish theology. But according to Rodkinson in the History of the Talmud, some of the Talmudic teachings may have permeated from and into other contemporary cultures (Gorfine 1984).

Talmudic thinkers were public teachers, expounders of the Law, popular lecturers. They wished to spread "ethical teachings" among the people in single, concise, pithy, pointed sentences, well adapted "to impress the minds and hearts, or in parables or legends illustrating certain moral duties and virtues." Their teachings did reach the Jewish masses and influenced their conduct of life. In fact, the Talmud was (and in Orthodox Jewish circles remains) "a guide for human conduct" (Gorfine 1984, p. 82).

A Guide to Conduct Toward Women

Some of the teachings about "human conduct" toward women in the Talmud are heartbreaking—and infuriating. Devorah Baron, the daughter of a rabbi at the beginning of the twentieth century, witnessed her father's ruling at home and, in her book *Stories*, describes what she saw (Baron 1984). One of her stories is entitled "Kritot" ("Bill of Divorce" in Hebrew) and is particularly sad. The Hebrew word Kritot has the same root as "Krita," meaning "cutting off" or "amputation." In this story, Baron writes that of all those brought to receive a ruling by her father (thieves and the like), the most afflicted were the women about to be sent away from their husband's house, according to a halakhic ritual. Women expelled in this way were known as women "divorced in the heart" because their husbands did not love them anymore which, according to Jewish Law, was a legitimate reason for banishment. This was so even if the "divorced in the heart" had done everything for her husband throughout many years of marriage; cooked, cleaned, washed his clothes, and gathered wood to make him a fire. None of this carried any weight. The woman was sent away, even if expulsion was tantamount to a death sentence as she had nowhere else to go.

Another group who could be sentenced to expulsion from the husband's house comprised women who, after 10 years of marriage, had not given birth. Barrenness, too, was a legitimate reason for divorce in Jewish Law (Haven 2007). No matter where the fertility problem lay (and in 40–50% of cases, it is known to lie with the man), the woman was always blamed. She was sent away, banished from her husband's house; and no one in the room protested because women were resigned to this ruling. As Rivka Gorfine notes in the introduction to Baron's stories, even if the rabbi himself believed the situation to be unfair, he proceeded with the divorce ceremony till the end (Baron 1984). This was Jewish Law. In the story "Family," a chance error that occurred while writing the document sufficed to invalidate the divorce, following which the woman returned home with her husband of 10 years—and became pregnant (Haven 2007).

Jewish Law (Regarding Women) in the 21st Century

According to some people, the role of women in traditional Judaism "has been grossly misrepresented and misunderstood," and the position of women in this tradition "is not nearly as lowly as many modern people think." (Haven 2007, p. 115). Christina Haven contends that the position of women in Halakhah (Jewish Law) that dates back to the biblical period "is in many ways better than the position of women under US civil law as recently as a century ago." She adds that many of the important feminist leaders of the twentieth century (Gloria Steinem, for example) are Jewish women, and suggests that this is no coincidence; because "the respect accorded to women in Jewish tradition was a part of their ethnic culture." Although Haven concedes that in traditional Judaism, women's obligations and responsibilities are "different" from men's, she immediately adds "but no less important. And, even in some ways, women's responsibilities are considered more important…" (Glaser 2021, p. 115). Yet where is the evidence? Gloria Steinem and other Jewish women became important feminist leaders in the twentieth century not because of the respect accorded to women in Jewish tradition "as a part of their ethnic culture," but because they rebelled against it.

This was also my personal experience growing up in a Jewish family during the second half of the twentieth century. Unambiguously, my brother was the important child. He was the good-looking one (I concur); he was smarter, nicer, more righteous and, overall, more successful. Of course, in many families, one child is considered more important than the other/s. However, while my brother was two years older than me, it was explicitly clear that the reason for his primacy was his sex. This superiority—as a boy—was a cultural motif that had further legitimacy in the extended Jewish community. For example, we both had a musical ear and could sing quite well, but my brother was allowed to join the synagogue choir, whereas I could not; because I was a girl. Since only men and boys were permitted on the main floor of the synagogue, I used to listen to the male-only choir rehearsals from the second floor, where women and girls—clearly second-class individuals—were allowed to be. As a result, I knew the religious songs by heart, but being a girl, had to sing quietly to myself. Girls and women were not allowed to sing in public.[16]

Generally, we girls had to internalize the fact that boys are the "important" people. We also realized early on in our lives that, someday, we were supposed to help the boys have children, and raise them. Morning prayers may best tell the whole story of men and women in the Jewish tradition: men thank God "for not making me a woman." Women thank God "for making me according to His will." I rebelled against what I was supposed to do and to be, just like Gloria Steinem and other important feminist leaders of the twentieth century, not because of traditional Jewish teachings, but in spite of them.

Orthodox Jewish politicians and rabbis, while recently answering the question of why neither of the two Haredi religious parties in Israel have even one woman member, explained that politics and the government is no place for women; precisely reiterating Haven's words above: "Women's obligations and responsibilities are different from men's…but no less important." And, "in some ways, women's responsibilities are considered more important…" (Glaser 2021). Indeed, an Orthodox Jewish woman is at home, conceiving and giving birth, dutifully following the first commandment in the Bible. She may also work to provide for the family, so that her husband can learn Torah for his entire life. But a woman's "more important" obligation and responsibility remain in her womb.

Biblical Teachings and the Lives of Women Today

Worldwide, mothers are overworked, underpaid, often lonely and made to feel guilty about everything from epidurals to bottle feeding. Fixing this is the unfinished work of feminism (Eliane Glaser). (Glaser 2021)

Some may argue that biblical and Talmudic teachings do not influence the lives of secular women today. But they do. Recently, for example, a successful pilot to evaluate whether women could serve as officers in the Armored Corps of the Israel Defense Forces was discontinued due to intervention by the Military Rabbinate in IDF decisions. Officers of the highest rank who were responsible for this pilot pointed out publicly—on TV—that the successful women officers in the pilot had performed the same tasks as many of the men, no less well and sometimes even better. Nevertheless, the four women who had attained the rank of officer were sent home with no further explanation.

A rabbi from a national religious party appeared on TV and offered the following argument against women's inclusion in the Armored Corps: "Who will marry these girls?" This line of reasoning may suffice to convince non-Orthodox but traditional believers, and even secular people, that their inclusion is a bad idea. For a woman's "duty" to marry and have children remains of highest priority in present-day Israel, among non-religious Jewish women as well.

---

[16] This continues in modern Israel. Women and girls in Orthodox Jewish communities are not allowed to sing in public; and this Jewish "tradition" sometimes permeates national events from which women find themselves excluded.

This is what the Bible—quite convincingly—has always taught and, unknowingly for many, still teaches. While many people may not believe in the Bible as God-given, biblical teachings about women and women's role still resonate with contemporary attitudes toward women, including women's beliefs about themselves. For example, Sarah Knott, the author of Mother, reminds us that, in the twentieth century "even the screen siren Elizabeth Taylor was 'a Woman at last' only once she had a baby…;" and observes that, even in the twenty-first century, "a 'Barren Woman' imagines herself like an empty museum, all pillars, porticoes and rotundas but not sanctuary." (Knott 2019, p. 35).

In a recent article in The Guardian, Eliane Glaser complains that the "perfect mother" has become "a cult" (Glaser 2021). But this "cult" is nothing new. As seen in this chapter, its roots can be found in a book written more than two millennia ago. Nevertheless, Knott's and Glaser's words are the best proof that, in the twenty-first century, biblical teachings about women and their role—for religious and non-believing women alike—persist.

3.5 Conclusions

"Be fertile and replenish the earth" is the first and most powerful commandment in the Bible. It is also the first written policy involving the womb. Nevertheless, while God had ordered humans to be fruitful, barrenness—the worst curse for a woman in the Bible—remains a central topic. Barrenness and God's intervention by miraculously opening the womb are a recurring motif in relation to mothers of heroic or important sons. Fertility is so crucial that even the most important women in the Bible, the four matriarchs, are barren. They are able to conceive only after God lifts the curse that "closed" their wombs. According to the Bible, for a woman, childlessness is worse than death. So much so, that in order to conceive, it is even acceptable to act as a prostitute and to practice deceit.

While the stories in the book of Genesis are considered to be an etiologic explanation of the world, such strong promotion of reproduction is strange since children arrive naturally after heterosexual intercourse. As many newborns in ancient times did not survive, it is plausible that new, powerful doctrines had to be developed to improve demographic outcomes; and, by present-day notions, they had to be marketed. Hence the biblical teaching—again and again—that a woman's role is to be with child; she is the recipient who will perpetuate a man's seed.

This was womb politics in the Bible. However, more than two millennia later, in the context of this book, women still internalize this role. To reproduce has remained a powerful commandment in the cultures descended from the three monotheistic religions; and continues to dictate women's lives until today. To be a woman with child remains—explicitly and implicitly—a social directive; childless women are—supposed to be—miserable and pitied. So much so that even in the twenty-first century, a woman's "destiny" may rely on her capability to reproduce. Infertility continues to be an insufferable condition for many women (see also Chap. 6). Finally, but by no means least, demographic whims and policies addressing the womb persist also in present times. In May 2021, for example, an article entitled "How do you convince people to have babies?" appeared on the BBC website (Hegarty 2021). The writer of this article is a modern "population correspondent" addressing demographic declines in China and the United States. The next chapter explores modern demography.

Acknowledgments I thank Dr. Ada Geva for her advice on biblical stories related to infertility. Any errors in this chapter are mine alone.

Notes

(1) The role of law—Open Knowledge Repository—World Bank Organization. https://openknowledge.worldbank.org/bitstream/handle/10986/25880/9781464809507_Ch03.pdf. Accessed 7 May 2021.
(2) If the global MMR falls to less than 70 deaths per 100,000 live births by 2030 (the SDG target), there will be 89,000 maternal deaths in 2030, and somewhere between 2 and 5 million deaths cumulatively between 2016 and 2030. https://data.unicef.org/topic/maternal-health/maternal-mortality/. Accessed 8 May 2021.
(3) https://www.mayoclinic.org›syc-20354317. Accessed 5 May 2025.
(4) https://www.thefreedictionary.com/barrenness.
(5) Infertility. Explanation by the Gesher Education Enterprise. Centre of Educational Technology. https://lib.cet.ac.il/pages/item.asp?item=12625. Accessed 5 May 2021.
(6) Coopersmith, Dina. Women in the Bible. www.aish.com/jl/b/women/Women_in_the_Bible_Rivka.html.
(7) Genesis, Chapter 25: 23. https://www.kingjamesbibleonline.org/.
(8) Genesis, Chapter 25: 24. https://www.kingjamesbibleonline.org/.
(9) Genesis, Chapter 29: 31. https://www.kingjamesbibleonline.org/.
(10) Judges, Chapter 13: 3, 5. https://www.kingjamesbibleonline.org/.
(11) Samuel I, Chapter 1: 11. https://www.kingjamesbibleonline.org/samuels-birth_bible/1:11.
(12) Genesis, Chapter 38: 7–10.

References

Baron, Devorah. 1984. *Family. Collected Stories*. Tel Aviv: Yachdav & Agudat Hasofrim (Hebrew).
Glaser, Elaine. 2021. Parent Trap: Why the Cult of the Perfect Mother has to End. *The Guardian* (18 May). https://amp.theguardian.com/lifeandstyle/2021/may/18/parent-trap-why-the-cult-of-the-perfect-mother-has-to-end.
Follet, Ken. 1989. *The Pillars of Earth*. London: MacMillan.
Gorfine, Rivka. 1984. Introduction. In *Collected Stories*, ed. Baron, Devorah. Tel Aviv: Yachdav & Agudat Hasofrim (Hebrew).
Greenblatt, Stephen. 2017. *Adam and Eve. The Story that Created Us*. London. Penguin.
Haven, Christine. 2007. *Conveyance of Eternal Love*. NY: Owl Creek Press.

Hegarty, Stephanie. 2021. *How Do You Convince People to have Babies*? (16 May). https://www.bbc.com/news/world-57112631.amp. Accessed 18 May 2021.

Knott, Sarah. 2019. *Mother. An Unconventional Story*. London: Random House.

Rodkinson, M.L.T. 1918 [1903]. *History of the Talmud. Babylonian Talmud*. http://www.sacred-texts.com/jud/t10/ht212.htm. Accessed 28 June 2019.

Witt, Emily. 2018 [2016]. *Future Sex*. London: Faber & Faber.

Chapter 4
Demography Wars

At whatever point of the spectrum – no babies or illegitimate babies or too many babies – women find themselves caught in a steel vice. (Jacqueline Rose 2019, p. 37)

The word "demography" is composed of two Greek words, "demos" meaning "people" and "graphy" meaning "science."[1] The term has been ascribed to a Belgian statistician, Achille Guillard, who coined it in 1855. According to historical accounts, however, the origins of modern demography are usually traced back to John Graunt's quantitative analyses of the "Bills of Mortality," published in 1662. Graunt's Bills of Mortality provided weekly lists of burials and baptisms in the parishes of London. He used these data to examine the sex ratio at birth and to estimate the population of London.[2] The simplest definition of demography, according to Peter McDonald and Emily Grundy, honorary demographers at The International Union for the Scientific Study of Population (IUSSP), is "the scientific study of human populations."[3],[1] Demography is concerned with the "numbering of the people" and with the understanding of population dynamics.[3] For demographers, a population is a group of individuals, who coexist at a point in time and share a characteristic, such as residence in the same geographical area. The age and sex structure of a population results from past trends in fertility, mortality, and migration.[2]

As noted in the previous chapter, the "numbering of people" appears as early as in the Bible, in God's very first commandment: "Be fertile and *replenish* the earth." This commandment is, in fact, the first *written* indication of the utilization of the womb for demographic purposes. Indeed, Orthodox Jews still follow this directive, giving birth to as many children as they can. This is the first evidence of the perception of

---

[1] The IUSSP is a permanent international organization, which scientifically considers the problems of population. Its mission is to promote the scientific study of population, encourage exchange between researchers around the globe, and stimulate interest in population issues. The Union was officially founded in 1928, in Paris, following the International Population Conference in Geneva in 1927. This was the first World Population Conference, organized by Margaret Sanger, stressing the crucial nature of the population problems and their influence on social, economic, and political situations. https://iussp.org/en/about/what-is-demography

F. Simonstein, *Womb Politics: A Short History of the Future of Human Reproduction*,
The International Library of Bioethics 99,
https://doi.org/10.1007/978-3-031-11654-4_3

the womb as a political tool; but policies to either increase or decrease the number of people in a population have been implemented throughout history. In the current Israeli–Palestinian conflict, for instance, the womb is a war tool, declared as such by both sides of the struggle. Utilization of the womb for demographic purposes has been known in other parts of the world, as well; notoriously in the twentieth century in China. In the Former Soviet Union, in Germany during the Third Reich, as well as in the United Sates and some other European countries, based on eugenics ideals (Simonstein 2004).

This chapter examines the womb as an instrument in demographic wars and asks whether and why women enroll, either willingly or unwillingly, in this scheme. First, the chapter gives a brief overview of the history of birth control and its discontents; it then explores the intervention of the law in demographics and describes current trends and societal determinants of fertility. It concludes by addressing the situation of women in demography actions.

4.1 Birth Control—And Its Discontents

In 1798, Thomas Malthus wrote An Essay on the Principle of Population, in which he posed the conundrum of geometrical population growth outstripping arithmetic expansion in resources. Malthus was an Anglican clergyman, who recommended late marriage and sexual abstinence as methods of birth control. After Malthus, some early 19th-century philosophers including Jeremy Bentham, Francis Place (he himself was the father of 15 children), and John Stuart Mill, suggested more pragmatic birth control methods such as coitus interruptus, vaginal barriers, and post-coital douching.[4] Robert Dale Owen, the son of a Scottish social reformer, helped spread these ideas in North America, and in 1832, a Massachusetts physician, Charles Knowlton, wrote The Fruits of Philosophy: or The Private Companion of Young Married People. According to historical accounts, although Knowlton's first edition of this short book was published anonymously, he was fined and imprisoned.[4] The Fruits of Philosophy appeared in England two years later and continued to be read for the next 50 years. In 1876, a Bristol publisher was prosecuted for selling it. However, the leader of Britain's National Secular Society and subsequently a Member of Parliament, Charles Bradlaugh, and Annie Besant reissued the pamphlet and provocatively notified the police. They were charged and tried by the public prosecutor, who claimed it to be "a dirty, filthy book," but the conviction was quashed on grounds of a faulty indictment.[4]

Nonetheless, according to historical accounts, the trial received wide publicity and, through the national press, "brought birth control onto the breakfast table of the English middle classes" at a time when, for economic reasons, they were eager to control their fertility. Furthermore, the Malthusian League, founded some years earlier by George Drysdale, began to attract wide public support. Similar leagues began in France, Germany, and The Netherlands, the latter opening the world's first family planning services, under Dr. Aletta Jacobs, in 1882.[4]

Women and Birth Control

Birth control became the object of a national, and ultimately global, social movement (see also Chap. 4) thanks to two women, Margaret Sanger in the United States and Marie Stopes in Britain. Both used the controversy surrounding birth control to draw attention to the issue. Sanger, a trained nurse, encountered miserable conditions in her work among the poor. She was inspired to take up her crusade after attending to a woman who was dying from a criminally induced abortion (Eig Jonathan 2014). In 1914, Sanger founded a magazine, *The Woman Rebel,* to challenge laws restricting the distribution of information on birth control. She was indicted and fled to Europe, but when she returned to stand trial in 1916, the charges against her were dropped. Later that year, she opened a family planning clinic in Brownsville, Brooklyn, New York, but the police immediately closed it, and Sanger was arrested and convicted on charges of "maintaining a public nuisance" (Eig Jonathan 2014). In Britain, the movement for birth control was led by Marie Stopes, the daughter of a middle-class Edinburgh family. She was one of the first women to obtain a doctorate in botany (from the University of Munich in 1904). In 1918 she published an appeal for sexual equality and fulfillment within marriage, *Married Love* that, at the time, was considered a radical text.[5] According to historic records, Margaret Sanger met Marie Stopes and persuaded her to add a chapter on birth control (Eig Jonathan 2014).

The existence of contraception and abortion throughout recorded history is clear evidence for a desire to control fertility under at least some circumstances (Sear et al. 2016). In the era of Sanger and Stopes, however, the term "birth control" was extremely problematic. It went against the Church and violated the perceived morality of the time, both in the United States and in England.[5] (Chesler 2011). After World War I, Sanger sought wider acceptance for the idea and substituted it with the more socially sounding term "family planning"—a move that was quite inventive then, because the Great Depression brought attention to collective needs (Chesler 2011, see Chap. 4). Sanger's advocacy emphasized the alleviation of poverty and overpopulation.

Stopes sought, in addition, to relieve women of the physical strain and risks of excessive childbearing. Her *Married Love* was followed by *Wise Parenthood* in 1918.[4] In 1921, Stopes opened a family planning clinic in Holloway, North London, the first in the country. It offered a free service to married women and also gathered data about contraception. In 1925, the clinic moved to Central London and others opened across the country. By 1930, other family planning organizations had been set up and they joined forces with Stopes to form the National Birth Control Council (later the Family Planning Association).[5]

In the United Sates, after many vicissitudes, a compromise was reached and family planning clinics were allowed on the condition that physicians were not involved in prescribing contraceptives. In 1936, a New York court, in a case known as *United States* v. *One Package of Japanese Pessaries,* ruled that contraceptives could be sent through the post if they were to be employed intelligently by conscientious physicians for saving life or promoting the well-being of their patients.[4]

Family Planning

Family planning was one of the first subjects to be investigated in demographic surveys. Fertility history and family planning data have remained the focus of many demographic surveys since the 1970s, for example, the World Fertility Survey. Presently, demography bears on the efforts of international agencies and national governments to promote family planning and improve health in the developing world. In the developed world, population growth has slowed, but low fertility and the reduction in death rates in old age are producing an increasingly aged population.[1]

Currently, family planning movements emphasize the right of the individual to determine family size as well as the potential contribution of family planning to national and global population problems.[4] Some methods of birth control, such as coitus interruptus and, in extreme cases, abortion, may involve no person other than the individual or the couple. Most methods, however, require manufacture, distribution, promotion, counseling and, in some cases, financial subsidy. In particular, social marketing programs, which adjust prices to people's needs, have allowed governments to make contraceptives available to large numbers of people, quickly and at affordable cost.[4]

Most of the changes that occurred in patterns of family planning took place before public family services were established and at considerable emotional and physical cost to many couples. By contrast, the majority of governments of contemporary Third World countries have established national family planning policies and actively encourage the use of public family services. The World Fertility Survey shows that more couples in developing countries desire small families than actually achieve their goals.[4]

Why small families? In a traditional agricultural society, children bring hope of economic rewards to their parents at an early stage by sharing in the work that is necessary to support the family, whereas in modern industrial societies, childcare and education require long years of heavy expenditure by parents. This switch in the cost of children may be the most important factor determining the adoption of family planning.That being said, the variables that encourage small families are still not fully understood; however, according to social and political studies, they include urbanization, educational and employment opportunities for women, and easy access to family planning services.[4]

Demography and the Law

The law, by defining marriage age, regulating medical practice, and controlling advertising and factors such as the employment of women, also affects many other variables that determine reproductive matters and the size of a family. Regarding controversial aspects of birth control, legal positions have oscillated, depending on circumstance and on government.[4] For example, the ruling on Roe v. Vade permitted legal abortions in the United States; but this ruling is now threatened by some right-wing governors (for further discussion on abortion, see Chap. 5). In the nineteenth century, the law was used as an assertion of extant morality. In the United States, for example,

Anthony Comstock lobbied to pass an Act for the Suppression of Trade and the Circulation of, Obscene Literature and Articles of Immoral Use. Anti-contraceptive and anti-sterilization clauses were added to the Napoleonic Code that applied to France and French colonies. In Britain, however, the law never specifically condemned contraception or sterilization, and Bradlaugh and Besant, who reissued the pamphlet *The Fruits of Philosophy* (see above), were accused under the Obscene Publications Act.[4]

In 1920, Lenin legalized abortion in the revolutionary Soviet Union as the right of every woman "to control her own body." He opposed the practice of contraception or abortion for purposes of regulating population growth. However, Lenin's successor, Joseph Stalin, adopted a pronatalist argument, in which population growth was seen as a stimulant to economic progress. As the threat of war intensified in Europe in the 1930s, Stalin promulgated coercive measures to increase Soviet population growth, including the banning of abortion despite its status as a woman's basic right.[6] In addition, the Nazi Third Reich "invaded the bedrooms of its citizens" before it moved its troops into the Sudetenland and Czechoslovakia. It forbade the display of contraceptives, which it condemned as the "by-product of the asphalt civilization."[6]

By contrast, the Proclamation of Teheran in 1968 (paragraph 16) states that "Parents have a basic human right to determine freely and responsibly the number and spacing of their children." This concept was written into Yugoslavia's constitution, and China officially made family planning an obligation for each citizen. U.S. courts interpreted the constitutional right of privacy to include birth control choices when the Comstock Act was finally overthrown in the cases of *Griswold* v. *Connecticut* (1965) and *Eisenstadt* v. *Baird* (1972). In Ireland, the case of Mary McGee (1973) reversed an Irish anti-contraceptive law of 1935, and in the Luigi deMarchi case in 1971, the Italian Supreme Court struck down the Fascist laws limiting the availability of contraception. At the other extreme, Singapore passed legislation removing certain tax credits from couples with three or more children.[4]

4.2 Present Trends in Demography

The human herd has been culled in the past by famine or plague. This time, we are culling ourselves; we are choosing to become fewer. Will our choice be permanent? The answer is: probably yes. (Adair Turner 2019)

The United Nations currently forecasts that the population will grow from 7 to 11 billion during this century, before leveling off after 2100. However, an increasing number of demographers around the world believe that the U.N. estimates are too high. They say that a more likely suggestion is that the planet's population will peak at around 9 billion sometime between 2040 and 2060, and will then start to decline. According to Bricker and Ibbitson (2019), by the end of the twenty-first century, we could be back to where we are right now, and steadily decreasing. Indeed, populations are already declining in about two dozen states around the world; by 2050, the number will have climbed to three dozen. Some of the richest places on earth are shedding people every year: Japan, Korea, Spain, Italy, and much of Eastern Europe.The really "big news," according to Bricker and Ibbitson, is that the largest developing nations are also about to grow smaller, as their own fertility rates come down.

The significance of the choices facing policymakers and individual families can be illustrated by reference to trends in family planning in the People's Republic of China (Clarke 2015). For a generation after the Revolution of 1949, national leaders maintained that a Communist economy could accommodate any rate of population growth, and family planning services, while available, were not emphasized. As a result of the rapid population growth in the 1950s and 1960s, however, the number of marriages in China each year soon exceeded, by 10,000,000, the number of fertile partnerships broken by death or by the onset of the woman's menopause.[4] In an attempt to stabilize the population, the Chinese government instituted a policy with the goal that 50% of rural couples and 80% of urban couples have only one child. In the first decade of the twenty-first century (Rosenberg 2018), however, the low birth rate and the increased size of China's aging population led to some relaxation of the one-child policy (Feng et al. 2016; Oskar and DeLong 2016).

Though governments have sometimes been able to increase the number of children couples are willing to have, through generous child care payments and other supports, they have never managed to bring fertility back up to the replacement level of, on average, 2.1 children per woman needed to sustain a population. Besides, such programs are extremely expensive and tend to be cut back during economic downturns. In addition to which it is arguably unethical for a government to try to convince a couple to have a child that they would otherwise not have had (Adair 2019). Still, some of those who fear the consequences of a diminishing population (such as fewer youngsters able to support an aging population) advocate government policies to increase the number of children per couple. Yet Bricker and Ibbitson, in the book *Empy Planet*, observe that the evidence suggests that this is futile. In their view, the "low-fertility trap" ensures that, once one or two children becomes the norm, it stays the norm. Couples no longer see having children as a duty to satisfy their obligation to their families or their God. Rather, they choose to raise a child as an act of personal fulfillment; and they are quickly fulfilled (Bricker and Ibbitson 2019).

Moreover, Bricker and Ibbitson claim that, within a few years, China will begin losing people. By the middle of this century, Brazil and Indonesia will follow suit. The authors contend that even India, soon to become the most populous nation on earth, will see its numbers stabilize in about a generation and then start to decline. Fertility rates remain sky-high in sub-Saharan Africa and parts of the Middle East, but even there, things are changing as young women obtain access to education and birth control. Moreover, Africa is likely to end its unchecked baby boom much sooner than the United Nation's demographers think (Bricker and Ibbitson 2019).

On the other hand, Burger and Delong argue that increased low-fertility incentives still need to be in place because if culture fails "to deliver fertility-limiting norms" to any major portion of society, fertility may rise. Nevertheless, they observe that some factors may keep fertility low; for example, "life comforts" that are "more attainable with fewer children." (Burger and DeLong 2016). Yet they find that, at very high levels of development in several wealthy countries, fertility levels are currently increasing. These increases seem to be due to institutional adjustments that increase gender equality, or reduce the relative costs of childbearing. This suggests, in their view, that it is not just distaste for larger families that is keeping fertility low, even in highly modernized contexts. It also suggests that a fertility uptick may already be underway (Burger and DeLong 2016).

Cultural Mechanisms of Human Fertility

Studying reproductive decision-making in humans rather than in animal models may offer the advantage that subjects can be asked about why they make the decisions they do. It seems that individuals can behave in ways that may increase or decrease fertility without conscious strategizing. Indeed, the evidence on the extent to which fertility decisions are consciously determined is mixed. According to Sear et al., fertility is "a complex phenomenon" as it is partly physiologically and partly behaviorally determined. Decades of research on human fertility has presented a clear picture of *how* fertility varies, including its dramatic decline over the last two centuries in most parts of the world. *Why* fertility varies, both between and within populations, however, is not so well understood (Sear et al. 2016).

Moreover, not only do cultural institutions (such as marriage and inheritance practices) influence fertility by acting as part of our socioecology, but cultural norms (such as breastfeeding practices, sexual behavior, and the acceptability of contraception) may play a more active role in explaining why fertility is so variable between individuals and populations, as they have the potential to change quite rapidly over time.For example, fertility decisions are influenced by both the physiological condition and behavioral strategies of the partners and parental investment decisions may include whether or not to invest in or continue investing in a particular child. Infanticide and abandonment have, evidently, both been common forms of disinvestment historically and cross-culturally, in addition to breastfeeding decisions and restricted sexual activity aimed at prolonging birth intervals (Sear et al. 2016). Yet results are inconsistent with a purely individualistic, rational-actor model of fertility and suggest that optimization of reproduction is driven partly by cultural dynamics beyond the individual (Colleran et al. 2014).

Cultural Norms

Norms and preferences are clearly an essential part of fertility decision-making in humans.
(Burger and DeLong 2016)

At present, the role of cultural norms, and how they spread, is central to the study of social demography and evolutionary demography (Burger and DeLong 2016). Models that are used for decision making in various fields, such as economics and public health, have begun to take cultural evolution into account, and a growing number also incorporate the modeling—verbal or mathematical—of the human ecosystem's expected coevolution with the spread of cultural practices (Creanza et al. 2017). Indeed, as humans are a social species, fertility is influenced by other individuals, including the availability and behavior of family and friends, wider social norms surrounding reproduction, and institutional factors that influence many aspects of fertility, family and work life, essentially providing the option set of strategies available to individuals within a social context. According to Sear et al., we may be particularly sensitive to the behavior of others because the availability of support to help us reproduce was vital for successful reproduction throughout our history. It may also pay to base reproductive behavior on observing the behavior of others, rather than using a trial-and-error approach. This is because births are relatively rare and costly events, leaving little opportunity to learn from trial and error (Sear et al. 2016). Nonetheless, the causal structure linking individual decisions to those of other people and to higher-level patterns remains poorly understood (Colleran 2016).

Many of the first models of cultural evolution drew explicit parallels between culture and genes by modifying concepts from theoretical population genetics and applying them to culture. Cultural patterns of transmission, innovation, random fluctuations, and selection are conceptually analogous to genetic processes of transmission, mutation, drift, and selection, and many of the mathematical techniques used to study genetics can be useful in the study of culture. However, these mathematical approaches had to be modified to account for the differences between genetic and cultural transmission (Colleran 2016). Indeed, the cultural transmission of traits is more complex than genetic transmission and may occur in short timescales, even within a single generation (Creanza et al. 2017). The fact that cultural traits need not conform to Mendelian inheritance is sufficient to produce complex evolutionary dynamics. For example, a child can acquire cultural traits not only from its parents (Mendelian vertical transmission) but also from nonparental adults (oblique) and peers (horizontal). Also, generally, the more common a cultural trait is in the population, the more likely it is for an individual to have the opportunity to acquire it through social learning (Creanza et al. 2017; Colleran 2016).

Social Learning: The Israeli Case

In Israel, for example, for any Jewish couple, having children—and more than one—is required and considered "a must." A Jewish married couple, from early on, may be badgered by relatives and friends with the question of whether they are expecting, to the extent that some women may enroll in IVF after only six months of unprotected intercourse. IVF is a booming industry in Israel, largely driven by the procreative max of Israeli society (see Chap. 6). This demand to have children, practically at all cost, is rooted in the first commandment in the Bible "Be fertile and replenish the earth" (see also Chap. 2). So much so that, among Orthodox Jews, if a couple remains childless after 10 years, the husband is allowed to divorce his wife and marry another woman. In addition is the imperative aimed at winning the longstanding conflict with the Palestinians through demographic means.[2] In turn, largely encouraged by their former leader Yasser Arafat, Palestinian women are also expected to make reproduction their main goal, for a demographic victory of the Palestinian cause over the Jewish population.

---

[2] Although it is usually said it is because of the 6 million of Jews murdered in the Holocaust.

4.3 Demography Policies and Women

Opting not to have children is a "selfish choice" (Pope Francis). (Gibson 2015)

Policies targeting the womb, to have either more, less, or no children, have undoubtedly had a huge impact on women. For instance, the application of the Chinese policies over time had an ironic effect on individual women: older women belonged to a generation that could not always obtain birth control services, and younger women were encouraged or, in some cases, even forced to abort pregnancies they wanted to keep.[4] Moreover, the one-child-only policy in China had the effect of baby girls being either aborted or abandoned, creating a major sex imbalance. However, while demographers and policy makers do care about this gender imbalance for men and about the excessive increase or decrease in population, the effects of demography policies on women have, generally, been neither mentioned nor discussed. For example, in the discussion about genetically enhancing future generations, which will require that all women who wish to give birth enrol in the IVF procedure, women are not taken into account (see Chap. 8). The womb bearers are apparently considered reproductive entities (vessels), which are utterly taken for granted.

Women's education has emerged as a central predictor of fertility decline (Snopkowski et al. 2016). In *Empty Planet*, Bricker and Ibbitson contend that the United Nation's present model does not consider the changes that are taking place in how people, *especially women*, are choosing to live their lives today. Furthermore, they observe that, in all successful economies where women are well educated and *free to choose*, a below-replacement fertility rate is the average result of diverse individual behavior. Some women (around 15–20%) choose to have no children; many choose to have one or two, and some have more. This happens also in urbanizing Latin America and even Africa, where "women are increasingly taking charge of their own destinies." Bricker and Ibbitson (2019) observe that these changes are leading to fewer children being born and, ultimately, to a shrinking world population.

Should women's new choices be accepted? Some of the current political leaders, such as Russian President Vladimir Putin, Turkish President Recep Tayyip Erdoğan, and Brazilian President Jair Bolsonaro, see population growth as a national imperative, and high fertility as "a female duty." (Adair 2019). Pope Francis has allegedly added his voice to this chorus, preaching that "opting not to have children is a 'selfish choice.'"(Gibson 2015). In response to these chauvinist claims, Adair Turner, *a former chair of the United Kingdom's Financial Services Authority, and chair of the Institute for New Economic Thinking*, states that "women's choices should be respected, although, on average, these choices will probably result in gradual population decline." (Adair 2019). Surely, providing girls with education and access to contraception and releasing them from the chauvinist demands of conservative religious or political leaders should be high priority (Snopkowski et al. 2016).

4.4   Conclusions

Explaining fertility change in humans is as crucial as it is difficult. Crucial, because it is the primary source of error for population forecasts, as well as a major determinant of future population structure, size, and growth rate. Difficult, because it is seemingly influenced by many social and environmental factors acting at multiple scales. Fertility responds to biology, economics, and technology, but it is commonly held that ideational factors of individual preferences and social norms are the primary determinants of the timing and amount of childbearing, especially at fairly low levels of fertility.

A consensus has not yet been reached on the range of birth control methods that society should offer. The right of couples to determine the number and spacing of their children is almost universally endorsed, whereas the possibility of coercive family planning is almost as widely condemned. Throughout the world, awareness of the advantages and disadvantages of specific methods of birth control, thoughtful judgments about ethics, and further evolution in medical and scientific knowledge will continue to be important to the welfare of the family, of individual countries, and of the entire globe.

In the context of womb politics, providing girls with education and access to contraception and releasing them from the chauvinist demands of conservative religious or political leaders would suffice and should be high priority. Women's education has emerged as a central predictor of fertility decline, but the many ways that education affects fertility have not been subject to detailed comparative investigation. Similarities across sites suggest that there are common elements in how education drives demographic transitions cross-culturally, but the differences suggest that local socioecologies also play an important role in the relationship between education and fertility decline. Deeper analysis of how human culture, human ecology, and the human environment coevolve is necessary for understanding historical and present dynamics, and for predicting future trends. These analyses will provide much-needed tools for the planning and direction of such dynamics. Humans' worldwide well-being and that of the ecosystem we live in depend on our ability to make such predictions and act accordingly.Mechanistic explanations of fertility decline are needed, at the very least, because there are multiple ways for individuals and populations to reach (or to miss) optimal solutions.

The next chapter focuses on the Advent of The Pill in the 1960s, the influential development that has affected present demography and family planning.

Notes

(1)   http://www.sociologydiscussion.com/demography/demography-meaning-scope-and-import
      ance-sociology/2932.
(2)   http://www.medicine.mcgill.ca/epidemiology/hanley/c609/material/DemographyEoB.pdf.
(3)   https://iussp.org/en/about/what-is-demography.

(4)   Social and political aspects of birth control. https://www.britannica.com/science/birth-control/
      Social-and-political-aspects-of-birth-control.
(5)   http://www.bbc.co.uk/history/historic_figures/stopes_marie_carmichael.shtml.
(6)   https://www.britannica.com/science/population-biology-and-anthropology/Malthus-and-his-
      successors#ref366943.

References

Bricker, Darrell, and John Ibbitson. 2019. *Empty Planet*. NY: Random House.
Chesler, E. 2011. A Woman with a Plan: The Real Story of Margaret Sanger. *Rewire News*. https://
    rewire.news/article/2011/11/03/a-woman-with-a-plan-the-real-story-of-margaret-sanger.
Colleran, Heidi. 2016. The Cultural Evolution of Fertility Decline. *Philosophical Transactions of
    the Royal Society B*. https://doi.org/10.1098/rstb.2015.0152.
Colleran, H., G. Jasienska, I. Nenko, A. Galbarczyk, and R. Mace. 2014. Community-Level Educa-
    tion Accelerates the Cultural Evolution of Fertility Decline. *Proceedings of the Royal Society B:
    Biological Sciences* 281. https://doi.org/10.1098/rspb.2013.2732.
Creanza, N., O. Kolodny, and M.W. Feldman. 2017. Cultural Evolutionary Theory: How Culture
    Evolves and Why it Matters. *Proceedings of the National Academy of Sciences of the United
    States of America* 114 (30): 7782–7789.
Clarke, Aileen. 2015. See How the One-Child Policy Changed China. *National Geographic*. https://
    www.nationalgeographic.com/news/2015/11/151113-datapoints-china-one-child-policy/.
Feng, Wang, Baochang Gu, and Yong Cai. 2016. *The End of China's One-Child Policy*. https://
    www.brookings.edu/articles/the-end-of-chinas-one-child-policy/.
Gibson, David. 2015. https://religionnews.com/2015/02/11/pope-francis-opting-not-children-sel
    fish-choice/.
Jonathan, Eig. 2014. *The Birth of the Pill*. London: McMillan.
Oskar, Burger, and John P. DeLong. 2016. What if Fertility Decline is Not Permanent? The Need for
    an Evolutionarily Informed Approach to Understanding Low Fertility. *Philosophical Transactions
    of the Royal Society B*. https://doi.org/10.1098/rstb.2015.0157.
Rose, Jacqueline. 2019. *Mothers. An Essay of Love and Cruelty*. London: Faber & Faber.
Rosenberg, M. 2018. *China One Child Policy Facts*. ThoughtCo. https://www.thoughtco.com/china-
    one-child-policy-facts-1434406.
Sear, R., D. Lawson, H. Kaplan, and M. Shenk. 2016. Understanding Variation in Human Fertility:
    What Can We Learn from Evolutionary Demography? *Philosophical Transactions of the Royal
    Society of London. Series B, Biological Sciences*. https://doi.org/10.1098/rstb.2015.0144.
Simonstein, F. 2004. *Self Evolution. The Ethics of Remaking Eden*. Tel Aviv: Yozmot (Chapter 2).
Snopkowski, K., M.C. Towner, M.K. Shenk, and H. Colleran. 2016. Pathways from Education
    to Fertility Decline: A Multi-site Comparative Study. *Philosophical Transactions of the Royal
    Society of London. Series B, Biological Sciences*. https://doi.org/10.1098/rstb.2015.0156.
Turner, Adair. (2019). *Two Cheers for a Declining Population*. https://www.fnlondon.com/amp/art
    icles/two-cheers-for-a-declining-population-20190130.

Chapter 5
The Advent of the Pill

For as long as men and women have been making babies they have also been trying not to.
(Jonathan Eig 2014, p. 7)

In the previous chapter, I explored how demography is influenced by fertility, birth control, and family planning. Yet the struggle to establish revolutionary ideas such as birth control and family planning is revealing, since it is thanks only to the pill that these ideas could succeed and thrive. I noted in Chap. 2 that since biblical times, barrenness has been regarded as a woman's curse.[1] Even today, for many women, infertility remains a curse, but throughout history, a pregnancy could be far worse—and certainly under dreadful living conditions. Poverty, for example, may create appalling conditions both for the newborn child and the mother, as well as for any existing siblings of the child. But poverty is not the only factor that can make a pregnancy unwelcome.

I had my first child when I was 18 years old. I was very young, but she was not an "accident." My partner was four years older, and we had been in a relationship for three years.[2] As young parents who wanted to devote ourselves to our baby daughter, we decided to postpone the arrival of a second child. I started on the pill. It was the 1970s and back then, I was completely unaware of being part of the first generation of women who could determine the course of their lives by choosing if, and when, to have a child. While researching the history of the pill to write this chapter, I learned how my fellow women, just a few years earlier, had not been as privileged as I was. A decade before then, the pill did not exist.

This chapter examines the history of the advent of the pill. It focuses on the life of women in the 1950s and what contraception and birth control meant in those days. It tells the story of the four heroes to whom we owe this development, explores the successes and difficulties of its marketing, and reviews what is happening today in the area of contraception.

---

[1] Probably before the Bible, but this is written evidence.

[2] We formally married—to stop my mother from crying because I was living in sin—when I was already five months pregnant.

© The Author(s), under exclusive license to Springer Nature Switzerland AG 2022
F. Simonstein, *Womb Politics: A Short History of the Future of Human Reproduction*,
The International Library of Bioethics 99,
https://doi.org/10.1007/978-3-031-11654-4_4

5.1   Women in the 1950s

Women in the 1950s were still expected to serve their men, and if the marriage failed, it was almost always the wife's fault. If a husband drank too much or had extramarital affairs, he was probably seeking refuge from an unpleasant home. If a woman failed to make her man happy, she was not trying hard enough. According to historical records, the 1950s were an especially challenging time for women. They risked being seen as outcasts if they graduated from college unmarried, if they got married and did not have children immediately, or if they had children but also wanted to work outside the home. To have a child out of wedlock was the greatest source of shame. Women in the 1950s tended to marry as soon as they could. A woman's role in life was to marry and have children, and to start at an early age. She was supposed to find satisfaction in serving her husband and her children. As Jonathan Eig puts it: "If she had desires of her own – be sexual, professional, or personal—she was expected to hold them in check, to wipe them out the same way she wiped germs from the kitchen counter or stains from the collars of her husband's white dress shirts" (Eig 2014, p. 9) while to rebel against these restrictions was to invite scorn and humiliation. Unmarried life was seen as empty and joyless, and women living it were to be pitied.

Nonetheless, there were signs that in the 1950s, women were ready to rebel against sexual and marital norms. In the 1950s, women were voting in roughly equal numbers to men for the first time in American history; and some forms of women's rebellion were taking root. When they married, or when they had children and wished not to have more, women turned to doctors, priests, and even newspaper columnists for advice, and did so without the same degree of shame that their mothers would have felt. "Contraception" was no longer a dirty word. Even Catholic women were exploring birth control, justifying it in their minds by thinking that this was, perhaps, one area where they knew better than the Church what was right and moral.Eig observes that most American women, with the exception of strict Catholics, accepted the idea of birth control, and most of them wished for a more convenient and effective method. For young women in the 1950s, fear of pregnancy was an unavoidable part of sex. A woman who was unmarried and pregnant was in terrible trouble. Single motherhood was not an option, at least not in the middle and upper classes. Abortion was illegal and underground abortions could be both dangerous and difficult to obtain, especially for those without money. Many women felt trapped—by their bodies, by their career options, by their contraceptive options, by pregnancy, and perhaps most of all, by their limited choices (Eig 2014).

According to Eig, by the fall of 1955, humans—and women in particular—were asserting themselves more than ever when it came to controlling their bodies and their lives. White, married, middle-class women were nesting in their suburban homes and making and raising children—lots of children—just as the stereotypes of the day said they should. But not all of these suburban housewives were happy about it. Then there were the women who were not white, married, middle class, or living in the suburbs. They had their own reasons to be dissatisfied. There were young

Black women moving from the South to the North and immigrant women arriving from distant countries, all exploring communities that offered new opportunities and perils. There were smart, young, unmarried women competing with men for places at law school and medical school. The Black women from the Deep South, the immigrant women, and the college women considering careers outside the home had something in common. Eig: "they recognized that the pursuit of opportunity required independence, and achieving that independence meant avoiding—or at least postponing—motherhood." (Eig 2014, p. 220).

5.2 Contraception and Birth Control

In the 1950s, women who married at 19 or 20 were done—or wished to be done—with babies by the time they were 30. This was not a novelty, however, since for as long as men and women have been making babies they had also been trying not to. Jonathan Eig reveals that the Ancient Egyptians made vaginal plugs out of crocodile dung. Aristotle recommended cedar oil and frankincense as spermicides. Casanova prescribed the use of half a lemon as a cervical cap. In the early 1950s, the most popular and effective form of birth control was the condom, a simple device that dated back to the mid-1500s, when the Italian doctor Gabrielle Fallopio tested a linen cloth made to fit the organs to prevent the spread of syphilis.

Since Fallopio, however, not much had changed. In the 1840s, condoms became cheaper and more widely available when the Goodyear Company began vulcanizing rubber. At the same time, crudely fitted cervical caps—an early form of diaphragm—began to appear. In the following century, little thought and even less effort had gone into innovation in the field.

Women, however, experimented with an array of contraceptive devices, but most of them did more harm than good. For example, during the 1930s, Celia Duel Mosher chronicled the sex lives of 45 women and found that 28 of them used contraception (Platoni 2010). It seems incredible to us today that the most popular form of contraception, at that time, was the antiseptic soap Lysol, which often caused inflammation and burning. The second most popular choice was the condom. Another was a "woman's shield," a device that was supposed to form a seal around the cervix and prevent semen from getting through, but these caps seldom fit properly. If the cap were too large, a woman might suffer cramping, ulceration, or infection; and if it were too small, pregnancy was likely. Most of the women in Mosher's study were affluent, with money and connections to visit doctors or to buy what they needed on the black market. In the days before antibiotics, these methods sometimes led to fatal infections of the uterus, ovaries, or fallopian tubes. Impoverished women often had no option other than an abortion, which could also have tragic results (Platoni 2010).

The first known description of an abortion appeared around 1500 BCE, in a medical text describing how a plant-fiber tampon coated with honey and crushed dates was used to end a pregnancy. In the nineteenth century, abortion rates rose dramatically. Women swallowed lye (caustic soda) and gunpowder, placed leeches inside their bodies, poked themselves with knitting needles, threw themselves down stairs, hammered their abdomen with brickbats, and swallowed potions. They were willing, in short, to risk serious side effects, arrest, and death rather than remain pregnant (Eig 2014).

In 1955, leaders in the birth control movement gathered in Puerto Rico for a conference sponsored by Planned Parenthood. During the conference, Planned Parenthood officials appealed to the World Health Organization to make child-spacing education part of its worldwide program of preventive medicine. They also asked the United Nations to recognize a woman's right to birth control as a basic human freedom. The United Nations rejected the proposal. The United States abstained from the vote.[1] Nevertheless, week after week, population control made more headlines, and with each headline came an increased sense that the problem was real, that the world's natural and economic resources would never keep up with the extraordinary growth in the number of people inhabiting the earth. Moreover, there was a growing sense, especially in America, that the baby boom was taking a psychological and emotional toll on the mothers responsible for raising those children. Ladies' Home Journal reported that women were working as much as 100 h a week for their families, even if they were in poor health. Was this really the best way to raise children? A magazine declared that this was a question that demanded national attention (Eig 2014).

5.3 Looking After the Pill

Among the key players in the development of the pill were two female activists: Margaret Sanger, who demanded a contraceptive that "women could eat like aspirin,"[2] and Katharine McCormick, who paid for the scientific research. Other activists were Gregory Pincus, a brilliant biologist who, at the time was a scientific outcast, and John Rock, a devout Catholic gynecologist who believed that a robust sex life made for a good marriage and argued tirelessly that the pill was a natural form of birth control.[2],[3] Sanger, McCormick, Pincus, and Rock, had, according to Jonathan Eig, something in common: they were rebels (Eig 2014). The next section focuses on their stories.

Margaret Sanger
Margaret Sanger was the founder of the birth control movement in the United States and an international leader in the field. She is credited with coining the term "*birth control.*"[4] She made her voice heard under the terrible outcomes of horrible abortions. Sanger started to seek a form of contraception that would enable women to have pleasurable sex, unafraid of the consequences for a woman, if she had sex—a pregnancy. Eig observes that, to many in 1950, that idea was as unthinkable "as putting a man on the moon." (Eig 2014, p. 3). Worse, it was dangerous. For what would happen, then, to the institutions of marriage and family? And what would happen to love? Indeed, if women had the power to control their own bodies, if they

had the ability to choose when and whether they got pregnant, many worried about what they would want next. But this is exactly what Margaret Sanger wanted. Sex without marriage. Sex without children, "Sex redesigned, re-engineered, made safe, and made limitless, for the pleasure of women." But in the first half of the twentieth century, this was considered dangerous. As Eig puts it:

> Two thousand years of Christianity and three hundred years of American Puritanism would come undone in an explosion of uncontrollable desire. Marriage vows would lose their meaning. The rules and roles of gender would be revocable. Birth control delivered by Science would do what the law so far had not; it would give women the chance to become equal partners with men. (Eig 2014, p. 3)

In 1956, a woman still had to be "shockingly bold" to admit in public that she liked having sex, especially if she was unmarried. Doctors still referred to sex as "the sex act," which, like the preparation of dinner, the ironing, and folding of laundry, was considered part of a married woman's household responsibilities. She performed the sex act either to make her husband happy or to propagate the species; she was not supposed to enjoy it. Indeed, women who craved sex too strongly were sometimes deemed in need of medical or psychiatric intervention (Eig 2014, p. 223). Yet amidst this grim reality, Margaret Sanger succeeded in popularizing the term "birth control" and almost single-handedly launched the movement for contraceptive rights in the United States. Women would never gain equality, she had argued, until they were freed from sexual servitude. Moreover, Sanger opened the nation's first birth control clinic in Brooklyn in 1916 and helped launch dozens more around the world.[4] In the end, however, instead of fighting for sexual liberation, she employed more pragmatic arguments, touting the importance of population control and family planning. She presented the notion of family planning to make the idea of contraception more palatable to public opinion, health providers, and politicians. With this euphemism she was able to obtain grants from wealthy friends and arrange meetings with world leaders—largely because she had taken the birth-control movement mainstream, arguing that contraception was a tool for economic growth and political stability (Eig 2014).

Katharine McCormick
Sanger carried the movement on her own; but by 1923, Katharine McCormick had assumed a central role. Katharine McCormick was a biologist and the second woman to graduate from MIT. She was vice president and treasurer of the National American Woman Suffrage Association and became vice president of the League of Women Voters after the 19th Amendment was ratified in 1920.[5] McCormick soon reached the conclusion that, without birth control, any woman might become a prisoner to her husband, a mere breeder. She asked herself: What was the point in fighting for women's rights and sending women to college. What was the point in asking women to fight for equality, when all they had to look forward to was getting pregnant? After her husband died, she became a millionaire with free reign over her wealth. Katharine donated more than $2 million (the equivalent of $23 million today) to research into the development of the contraceptive pill.[5]

McCormick helped Sanger open the nation's first legal birth-control clinic in Brooklyn. Known as the Clinical Research Bureau, it stayed on the right side of the law by positioning itself as a center for the study—not the distribution—of contraception. The clinic did distribute contraception, though, and it quickly ran out. Demand far exceeded supply. Diaphragms were routinely smuggled into the country from Canada, but this was not enough. Nevertheless, after decades of work, the contraceptive devices available in these clinics—condoms and cervical caps, mostly—remained ineffective, impractical, or difficult to obtain. Eig: "It was like Sanger [and McCormick] had been teaching starving people about nutrition without giving them anything healthy to eat." (Eig 2014, p. 230).

Gregory Pincus

At this point, Sanger approached Gregory Pincus, a biologist and perhaps the world's leading expert in mammalian reproduction. In the 1930s, at the start of his career, he had attempted to breed rabbits in Petri dishes using much the same technology that, decades later, would lead to in vitro fertilization for humans. He claimed that a new age of human reproduction was on the horizon, one in which men and women would soon employ modern methods to control the process of making babies. Science would lead the way. Americans were not yet ready to hear such things. According to historical records, the press compared Pincus to Victor Frankenstein, the fictional scientist, who tried to conjure life but accidentally created a monster. Harvard denied Pincus tenure, and no other university would hire him. He was deemed dangerous. When no other job arrived, he moved to Worcester, Massachusetts, for a low-paying, low-rank position as a researcher for Clark University. Pincus worked in a basement lab in lousy conditions for serious research. Since the university did not provide him with a proper laboratory, Pincus and a colleague launched their own scientific center. They founded the Worcester Foundation for Experimental Biology, went door to door asking for donations, and bought an old house where Pincus set up a lab in the garage.[6]

Sanger explained to Pincus that she was looking for an inexpensive, easy to use, and completely foolproof method of contraception, preferably a pill. It should be something a woman could swallow every morning, with or without the consent of the man with whom she was sleeping; something that would make sexual intercourse spontaneous, with no forethought or messy fumbling, no sacrifice of pleasure; something that would not affect a woman's fertility if she wished to have children later on in life; something that was 100% effective. At that time, however, this was considered dirty, disreputable work. The technology was not there; and even if it somehow could be done, there would be no point. Anti-birth control laws were still in place in 30 states and the federal government. So why go to the trouble of making a pill that no drug company would dare to manufacture and no doctor would prescribe? Yet Pincus had been an outcast from the scientific establishment, rejected as a radical by Harvard, humiliated in the press, and left with no choice but to conduct his varied and oftentimes controversial experiments in a converted garage. Nevertheless, according to Jonathan Eig, "he radiated confidence as if he knew the world would one day recognize his brilliance." (Eig 2014, p. 2).

Pincus knew, however, that one of the hardest parts of the process would be the large-scale human trials necessary for approval by the U.S. Food and Drug Administration (FDA). He was a scientist, not a clinical physician, and was barred from conducting human trials. What is more, significant legal restrictions on birth control devices made testing the drug virtually impossible. As it happens, Pincus met an old acquaintance, Dr. John Rock, at a medical conference in the early 1950s. Rock was already testing the hormone progesterone—the same hormone Pincus was testing as a contraceptive in rats—on his infertile female patients. To Pincus's surprise, John Rock had crossed the great divide between animal and human testing. Therefore, Pincus asked Rock to collaborate on human trials for the pill.[6] John Rock agreed to work on the contraceptive pill project.

John Rock

Rock seemed an unlikely choice because he was a highly-regarded obstetrician and gynecologist and a devout Roman Catholic. He was a ground-breaking infertility specialist, who devoted much of his career to helping women with fertility problems to conceive. But in the course of his practice, Rock had also witnessed the suffering women endured from unwanted pregnancies. Rock had seen collapsed wombs, premature aging, and desperation caused by too many mouths to feed. The experiences of his patients had a profound impact on him. Despite his faithful Catholicism and the Church's opposition to contraceptives, Rock came to support contraception within the confines of marriage. Although he never went as far as to endorse birth control purely as a woman's right, Rock believed in the power of birth control to stem poverty and to prevent medical problems associated with pregnancy. As a result, John Rock agreed to work with Pincus on the controversial project to create a "magic pill" contraceptive.[7]

As part of the infertility research at his clinic, Rock was able to conduct the first human trials for the pill in Boston, sidestepping the rigid Massachusetts anti-birth control law. Although a Catholic, Rock had already put his reputation on the line in 1931 by signing a petition, with 15 other prominent Boston physicians, urging the repeal of the Massachusetts law prohibiting the sale of contraceptives. Risking excommunication, he was the only Catholic doctor to make the stand. After the Catholic Church approved of the "rhythm method" in 1936,[3] Rock was the first doctor to open a rhythm clinic in Boston. There, he taught Catholic women how to use the only birth control method permitted by their Church. In addition, as a professor of obstetrics and gynecology at Harvard Medical School in the 1940s, Rock taught his students about birth control, something unheard of in medical schools at the time. In 1949, he coauthored a book, Voluntary Parenthood, explaining birth control methods for the general reader. By the time Gregory Pincus approached Rock in the

---

[3] The rhythm method is a form of natural family planning. To use the rhythm method, a woman tracks her menstrual history to predict when she will ovulate. This helps her determine when she is most likely to conceive. If she is hoping to get pregnant, she can use the rhythm method to determine the best days on which to have sex. Similarly, if she wishes to avoid pregnancy, she can use the rhythm method to determine which days to avoid unprotected sex. https://www.mayoclinic.org/tests-procedures/rhythm-method/about/pac-20390918.

early 1950s about the pill trials, Rock had also come to believe in the need for world population control.[7]

5.4   The Pill Trials

At the same time as Pincus had been giving a synthetic version of the hormone progesterone to rabbits and rats to inhibit ovulation, Rock was giving women the hormone to enable them to become pregnant. Rock worked with women who had no identifiable cause of infertility, but were still unable to conceive a child, placing these patients on a daily regimen of progesterone and estrogen for several months. He theorized that the drug would allow their bodies to "rest" from ovulation. Then, after stopping treatment, his hope was that the reproductive organs would "rebound" more vigorously and enable his patients to conceive.

Rock's instincts proved correct. After he administered the therapy to 80 patients, 13 of them conceived within four months of finishing the hormone treatments. In the nascent field of infertility treatment, statistics such as these were considered remarkable.[6] When Rock reported his findings, the medical world took immediate notice of what it called the "Rock Rebound." But few were interested in the most striking aspect of the experiment—the suspension of ovulation with the use of hormones.Under the guise of fertility research, Pincus had found a way to test the contraceptive powers of progesterone on women. Rock was intrigued by Pincus's experiments with progesterone alone, and agreed to test just the single hormone on his patients. Although Pincus and Rock camouflaged the true purpose of their study, the tests would be historic—the first human trials of an oral contraceptive.[6]

In 1954, Rock began his first tests of synthetic oral progesterone on a group of 50 infertility patients at his clinics. Pincus suggested that Rock adopt a 20-day regime that would stop ovulation and still allow women to menstruate every month. Pincus hoped that, with this regimen, the drug would be viewed as not interfering with a woman's normal reproductive functions. Rock jumped at the idea. Since this modified regimen mimicked the reproductive cycle, Rock believed the Catholic Church might consider the process "natural"—and therefore an acceptable form of birth control.The result was that not one of the 50 women ovulated during their time on the oral progesterone. Moreover, the oral contraceptive was not only effective, but the effects of the drug were temporary, thus eliminating any fear that the pill would have a permanent sterilizing effect.[6]In early 1956, Rock told the world about his clinical trials at a conference of scientists involved in hormone research. Although he avoided any direct discussion of the drug as a deliberate contraceptive, everyone listening knew he was talking about a pill that could control women's fertility. Moreover, in the 1960s, Rock became the pill's chief promoter and chief publicist. He became the face of the pill. He appeared regularly in Good Housekeeping magazine.[6] Although Pope Paul VI, in 1968, finally published a powerful ban against the pill,[8] John Rock, as a Catholic, did an enormous amount to encourage women to take the pill.[3]

Marketing the Pill

The pill had to be controversial. It was mostly untested and firmly opposed by the Catholic Church. By the 1950s, Roman Catholics made up 25% of the American population. And the drug companies were very scared that if they produced and marketed a birth control pill, not only would Catholics not buy the pill, but they would boycott all the other products made by that company.[3] Moreover, the Comstock Law, passed in the United States in 1873, was part of a campaign for legislating public morality in the US, intended to stop the trade in "obscene literature" and "immoral articles," which included birth control devices and information on such devices (Lewis 2019).

In 1938, the federal ban on birth control was lifted, but, in 1958, astonishingly, 17 states had laws banning the sale, distribution, or advertisement of contraception. In one state, it was a crime "to use any drug, medicinal article or instrument for the purpose of preventing conception." In another, it was a felony, "to exhibit, sell, prescribe, provide, or give out information" about contraceptives (Eig 2014, p. 276). Nonetheless, there were calls for the government not only to accept contraception but to step in and regulate it. Worthless products were sold, and quacks performed unsafe abortions. Furthermore, the pill was a drug that represented a potential goldmine to the company that marketed it first. This company was Searle. They quickly understood that this was a medicine women would take more often than either aspirin or penicillin; a pill they would take every day, possibly for years, in sickness and in health.[3] If it worked, if it won approval, if it did not make women sick, and if it became popular or, at least, socially acceptable, millions of women all over the world might each consume 240 tablets a year at a price of about 50 cents a pill. The numbers were mind-boggling.

Searle faced difficult questions, however: for example, what were the rules for testing a pill for healthy people? How far did a company have to go to prove the safety of such a product? Was one year of testing enough to measure long-term effects? Five? Ten? There were risks, but the rewards for this drug, in particular, were like no other. Jonathan Eig:

> This was a pill to be used to treat a healthy person and for long-term use. This was a drug that had the chance to make money, change lives, change the culture, and combat massive health problems such as hunger, poverty, and overcrowding… Moreover, childbirth was dangerous, too, especially for women who were sick, weak, or starving. (Eig 2014, p. 255)

There was no way to measure how many lives might be saved by a reliable contraceptive, but even without a measure, that data had to be factored into analysis of the dug's risks.Nevertheless, Searle's application to the FDA in 1957, for the drug Enovid, made no mention of contraception: amenorrhea, dysmenorrhea, and menorrhagia were the menstrual problems Enovid was said to combat. On June 10, 1957, the FDA approved the sale of Enovid for infertility and menstrual irregularities. The brand approved in England at about the same time was Enavid. Within two years, 500,000 women were getting prescriptions for the new drug. More women appeared to have developed menstrual disorders overnight.[3]

The pill was being prescribed everywhere because everyone knew that the real effect of the pill was to suppress ovulation. Searle stepped up to meet the growing demand for contraceptives, confident that the law would find a way to keep pace with the rapid cultural changes taking over throughout the United States. Suddenly, Searle saw the pill, not as a public relations problem, but as a potential money maker.[9] Searle decided to apply for FDA approval of the drug as a contraceptive, and John Rock suggested that, for the application, the company use phrases such as "child spacing," "postponement of pregnancy," and "suppression of ovulation," rather than "contraception" and "birth control." Searle would settle eventually on "family planning" as its euphemism of choice (Eig 2014, p. 278).

5.5 The Pill at Last

On July 23, 1959, Searle asked the FDA to approve Enovid for birth control. Ten months later, on May 9, 1960, the FDA approved the world's first commercially produced birth control bill—Enovid-10, made by the Searle Company.[10],[11] When Enovid officially came on the market in 1960 as a contraceptive, the response was astonishing. In less than two years, 1.2 million women were on the pill. By 1965, over 5 million women were using it. By the late 1960s, seven manufacturers were producing oral contraceptives, and in 1968, annual pill sales hit $150 million. World-wide, more than 12 million women were taking the pill.[9] Despite the fact that the original pill contained very high doses of estrogen and progesterone, causing an array of side effects, women preferred it to other methods such as the diaphragm, condoms, and douches. Douches were not very effective. Condoms required the cooperation of a partner and reduced pleasure. Diaphragms were awkward, required a lot of care, and took the spontaneity out of sex. Many women were willing to put up with nausea, bloating, weight gain and other side effects in exchange for an easy and practically foolproof birth control method that separated contraception from the act of sex.[9]

As the pill's popularity grew, however, so did concern over the social impact of an oral contraceptive. U.S. News and World Report warned about sexual anarchy. While some saw the pill as the decline of Western civilization and others saw it merely as shoring up American civilization, they shared the idea that extramarital sex was a bad thing. And whether they thought the pill would contribute to it or not, both conservatives and liberals tended to agree that women should not be promiscuous.[3] According to historian Andrea Tone, this was "the ultimate double standard," because in the late 1950s, condoms were freely available "and you didn't see social commentators up in arms about how condoms in the 1950s would increase male promiscuity; so female virtue is held up to a much higher standard."[3] Indeed, the pill was revolutionary on this front, giving some people plenty to fear. In a 1968 Readers Digest article, for example, Jonathan Eig cites author Pearl Buck saying: "Everyone knows what the pill is. It is a small object—yet its potential effect upon our society may be even more devastating than the nuclear bomb." According to Eig, Buck's argument seemed to be informed by a hysteria that sex without *why* would spell the end of civilization. For these people, the so-called sexual revolution was to blame for modern relaxed views on sex practices (Eig 2014).

The pill was only one factor. In the 1960s, American society was already beginning to change.[3] Researchers have noted sweeping changes in public perceptions of sex that began in the 1960s. A study published in 2015 examined American attitudes toward sex from the 1970s to the 2010s, and concluded that between those decades, Americans became more accepting of non-marital sex (Ambrosino 2019).

In the autumn of 1966, Margaret Sanger died at the age of 87. She had lived long enough to see her dream fulfilled, and the Comstock laws overturned.[4] Her scientist, Gregory Pincus, died a year later from over-exposure to toxic chemicals in the lab. Katharine McCormick died next, at 92. Only John Rock, the Catholic doctor, lived long enough to see the pill's full impact on American society.

Women After the Advent of the Pill

According to historical records, in 1959, the so-called baby boom was underway, and many women had already seen enough of it. By 1960, the baby boom was taking its toll. Mothers who had four children by the time they were 25 still faced another 15 to 20 fertile years ahead of them. Women wanted the pill and wanted it now. All they needed to do was to find a doctor who was willing to prescribe Enovid for menstrual regulation. Although it was not yet officially recognized as birth control, more than 500 women were taking the pill. For women across the country, the contraceptive pill was liberating; it allowed them to pursue careers, fueled the feminist and pro-choice movements, and encouraged more open attitudes toward sex.[3] The oral contraceptive gave women highly effective control over their fertility.

As the 1960s progressed, the Women's Liberation Movement gained momentum alongside the civil rights and anti-war movements. It was a time of change, especially for women. For the very first time, women could be free to enjoy sex, without the fear of pregnancy hanging over their heads. With almost 100% fertility control, women were able to postpone having children or to space births to pursue a career or a degree that had never been possible prior to the pill. It was a change toward what people in the business call a contraceptive mentality; a mentality that assumes that people plan their reproductive lives.[11],[3].

Although popular culture had glorified the image of the happy homemaker, in reality, vast numbers of American women worked outside the home. The female employment rate had dipped after World War II, but by 1954, more women were in the workforce than at the height of the war. Most women worked in low-paid jobs such as teaching, nursing, waitressing, and secretarial or factory work. Although women were able to enter professional fields thanks to the Civil Rights Act of 1972,

[4] There may be controversy over Sanger's support for eugenics. Yet, during the first part of the twentieth century, eugenics was regarded as a "scientific" theory widely accepted worldwide. Even Lionel Penrose, who is considered the "father" of Modern Genetics, changed his title from Professor of Eugenics to Professor of Genetics, during the 1950s, because of the Nazi connotation (Frida Simonstein, 2004, Remaking Humans. The Ethics of Self-Evolution. Yozmot).

which prohibited employment and educational discrimination, the pill also played a significant role.[11]

Within a few years, half of all women of childbearing age were on the pill. Being on the pill was the "fashionable thing" to do. Thanks to the pill, women could postpone pregnancy, finish college, go to law school and medical school, apply for jobs, and could take leading positions in government and the antiwar movement and in the fight for equal rights. Women became lawyers because law firms no longer had to worry that the woman would get pregnant in the middle of a big case. Women became doctors because they could space their children so that they had time to do internships and residencies. Moreover, women did not seem to be concerned "whether they got an MRS degree or not." It was revolutionary.[3]

In 1970, women comprised 10% of first-year law students and 4% of business school students. Ten years later, those numbers jumped to 36 and 38% respectively. Research has shown that the pill had a direct effect. In states that lowered the age of consent for contraception from 21 to 18, women were more likely to enroll in graduate school and postpone marriage. In Japan, however, where abortion rates were the highest in the world at the time, the government refused to approve the pill for decades, for fear that it might promote promiscuity. Only in 1999, after the government approved Viagra, did Japan make birth control legal (Eig 2014).

Surely, the pill did more for the equality of women than any other single factor, certainly in the twentieth century. My own experience is that, thanks to the pill, I could avoid having more children—after giving birth to a girl and a boy—and could go to university. Indeed, for the first time in history, women began to see themselves as economically self-sustainable units, which was one of the most profound changes. It is estimated that 80% of all American women born since 1945 have taken the pill. Thus, it is impossible to understand the history of modern women without thinking about what the pill did for women; as well as what the pill did to women.[12]

Backlash Against the Pill

When the pill came on the market in 1960, it was enthusiastically embraced by the medical profession and the public. By the late 1960s, however, thousands of women were complaining to their physicians about side effects. Earlier, during a preliminary study performed in Puerto Rico, three women had died while participating in the trial. They were never autopsied, and the cause of death remained unknown, but in the US, grim news began to filter through the medical community—the pill could kill. By the end of the decade, after a crisis over the drug Thalidomide (that was prescribed for morning sickness and caused birth defects) and increasing reports of potential health risks from the pill, confidence in the drug was receding. In 1969, concerns came to a head with the publication of The Doctor's Case Against the Pill. In this book, medical journalist Barbara Seaman combined the testimony of physicians, medical researchers, and women who had used oral contraceptives to build a case against the safety of the pill and to indict the medical-pharmaceutical establishment that had marketed it. U.S. Senator Gaylord Nelson, who was in the midst of conducting hearings on the pharmaceutical industry, investigating abuses in the use of antibiotics, barbiturates and tranquilizers, decided to take on the birth control pill next.[13]

In January 1970, experts assembled in the stately Senate chamber and began giving testimony on the hazards of the pill. Young women, members of the radical collective D.C. Women's Liberation, were in the audience listening to the experts. They had come to the hearings because they had all taken the pill at one time or another and had experienced side effects. As they heard the experts—one male witness after another describing serious health risks—they were furious that not a single woman who had taken the pill had been brought to testify. At the hearings, when one expert said that estrogen causes cancer, the women spectators began hurling questions at the men on the dais: "Why are you using women as guinea pigs?" and "Why are you letting the drug companies murder us for their profit and convenience?"[11],[13]

The narrator of the film about the pill provides a telling answer to these questions:

> It must be admitted that women make superb guinea pigs. They don't cost anything, they feed themselves, they clean their own cages, pay for their own pills, and remunerate the clinical observer.[12]

At this point, feminists saw the pill as yet another example of patriarchal control over women's lives. They decided to protest the structure of the hearings and the men leading them, in addition to speaking out about the medical dangers of the pill. An estimated 87% of women between the ages of 21 and 45 followed the hearings, as a result of which 18% quit taking the oral contraceptive. However, a few years later, prescription rates rebounded, and the number of users in the United States peaked at approximately 19 million.[11],5,[13] Why? Simply because diaphragms, condoms, and IUDs did not cause nausea or other side effects, but did not always prevent a pregnancy. These methods had high failure rates, and pregnancy came with its own list of side effects (including preeclampsia, diabetes, hypertension, and heart attack). In the end, the physical and emotional toll of nausea and bloating were nothing compared to the physical and emotional toll of an unwanted pregnancy; and for some women, even the long-term risk of cancer might pale compared to the dangers of pregnancy or abortion. As Eig notes: "to analyze the risks of the birth control pill effectively, one had to factor in the complications for women not using it." (Eig 2014, p. 292).

---

5 Interestingly, the real impact of the hearings was not on pill usage, but on the nascent consumer health movement. For the first time, D.C. Women's Liberation succeeded in making informed consent a national issue. In the aftermath of the hearings, the U.S. government required the pharmaceutical industry to include a patient information sheet with complete information on side effects in every package of birth-control pills sold. The growing women's movement was prompting women to assert control over their bodies, and in doing so, it forever changed the way Americans take prescription medications.

5.6 The Pill Today

Today, more than 100 million women are on the pill. It is the most common form of contraception in Europe, Australia, and New Zealand, the second most popular in Africa, Latin America, and North America, and the third most popular in Asia (Campo-Engelstein 2019). The original Enovid pill contained 10 mg of progesterone and 15 mg of estrogen to prevent ovulation. Later, however, researchers would learn that lower doses would suffice. Searle then applied for FDA approval of a version of Enovid that contained only 1 mg of estrogen and either 5 mg or 2.5 mg of progesterone. The lower dose pills caused far fewer uncomfortable side effects and were cheaper to manufacture, making the pill even more profitable for the pharmaceutical company. As a result of the Senate hearings, pharmaceutical companies lowered dosages even further. In the 1980s, the high-dosage 10-mg pill was removed from the market.[11]

Over the past two decades, the dangers of sexually transmitted diseases and AIDS have led to increased reliance on barrier methods of contraception; however, the pill remains the most popular reversible contraceptive in the UK and the USA, in spite of the various health scares since its invention in the early 1950s.[10] Nevertheless, side effects of oral contraceptives remain. These include intermenstrual spotting, nausea, breast tenderness, headaches and migraine (Migraine and the Contraceptive Pill, n.d.), weight gain (Lopez et al. 2016), mood changes, missed periods, decreased libido (Castelman 2014), vaginal discharge, changes to eyesight for those using contact lenses (Smith 2018). The pill can increase the risk of cardiovascular problems, such as blood clots, stroke, or heart attack[14] (Tzankova et al. 2010). Birth control pills have also been associated with an increase in blood pressure, benign liver tumors, and some types of cancer.[15] It is estimated that, overall, the risk of developing a serious blood clot is approximately 1/10,000 and the risk of developing a heart attack or stroke is approximately 1–5/100,000. However, only a small fraction of these cases are fatal. In comparison, approximately one out of every 10,000 women giving birth in the United States will die from a complication. These risks have not been eliminated because they are linked to hormone exposure and exist with pregnancy as well.[16] Moreover, today, the debate is not over the safety of the pill, but over the question of whether it should remain a prescription drug or become available over the counter.[11],[10]

Contraception Today

Today, the terms family planning and contraception are used interchangeably, for example, the WHO, in an article in 2018, indicates that "family planning/contraception" reduces the need for abortion, in particular unsafe abortion and reinforces people's rights to determine the number and spacing of their children. This is achieved "through use of contraceptive methods and the treatment of infertility." In addition, this article maintains that by preventing unintended pregnancy, "family planning /contraception" prevents deaths of mothers and children (WHO 2018). It is written in parenthesis, however, that the fact sheet focuses on contraception.

Furthermore, the WHO fact sheet claims that the promotion of family planning—and ensuring access to preferred contraceptive methods for women and couples—"is essential to securing the well-being and autonomy of women, while supporting the health and development of communities." This WHO publication also remarks that by reducing rates of unintended pregnancies, family planning also reduces the need for unsafe abortion (WHO 2018).

These statements by the WHO in the second decade of the twenty-first century *precisely* follow the claims made by Sanger at the beginning of the twentieth century. In addition, the WHO explains today that a woman's ability to choose if and when to become pregnant has a direct impact on her health and well-being. The WHO clarifies that family planning allows spacing of pregnancies and can delay pregnancies in young women that increase risk of health problems and death from early childbearing. Family planning, according to the WHO, prevents unintended pregnancies, including those of older women, who face increased pregnancy-related risks. It also enables women to limit the size of their families, if they so wish. Finally, the WHO publication remarks that evidence suggests that women who have more than four children are at increased risk of maternal mortality (WHO 2018).

Moreover, these days, researchers on contraceptives, freely and unapologetically, observe that in addition to the benefits to female health, family planning provides women with "an opportunity to pursue an education and/or employment, generating confidence and economic independence." (Kirtane et al. 2019). Indeed, the impact of female contraceptives on global good cannot be underestimated. So much so that a popular writer in 1968 ranked the importance of the pill alongside the discovery of fire and the development of tool-making. Twenty-five years later, the leading British weekly, The Economist, listed the pill as one of the seven wonders of the modern world. Indeed, for more than 40 years, more people have taken it than any other prescribed medicine (Wang et al. 2016). Margaret Sanger's revolutionary, "dangerous," and illegal ideas had come true.

5.7 Present Trends in Contraception

Several methods of hormonal contraception exist, including subcutaneous implants, intrauterine devices, vaginal rings, transdermal patches, injectables, and oral pills. Injectable formulations contain poorly soluble drug microcrystals that slowly dissolve in extracellular fluid and provide sustained serum concentrations for ~3 months. Shorter-term protection (~1 month) can be obtained with vaginal rings or transdermal patches (Ortho Evra). Implantable devices are polymeric systems that can provide drug release up to ~3 years, after which they are surgically removed. Several intrauterine hormonal devices are available, which provide protection for 3–6 years[17] (Kirtane et al. 2019).

Tablets have the shortest duration and need to be taken daily. Another option for hormonal contraceptives is the extended-cycle pill. It contains the same hormones as other birth-control pills, but the hormones are taken in a longer cycle. That reduces the number of menstrual periods from 13 per year to only four. That means that a woman who takes this pill will menstruate only once each season.[18] Microneedles are also being developed as a pain-free means of administering long-term contraceptives. Nevertheless, daily oral pills are favored by a sizeable fraction of the population, possibly because of their ease of use, opportunity for self-administration, and rapid resumption of fertility on discontinuation (Kirtane et al. 2019).

If the pill is used consistently by 1000 women, one of them will become pregnant after one year. In reality, many women may either forget, may take it at the wrong time of day, or delay starting a new packet after the last one is finished. Missing or delaying pills increases the risk of ovulation, fertilization, and pregnancy. Thus, taking "typical" use into consideration, up to 5–9% of pill users per year will become pregnant[16] (Smith 2018; Kirtane et al. 2019). Indeed, the effectiveness of oral contraception is compromised because of a lack of patient adherence, leading to unplanned pregnancies. A multinational survey has revealed that over a 3-month interval, nearly 40–50% of women missed at least one dose. A similar percentage of women reported having taken the medication at the wrong time. Therefore, to improve patient adherence, an oral contraceptive that is administered once a month has been developed. Kirtane et al. (2019) defended the development of these technologies as underscoring "the value long-acting contraceptives add to society".

"Women's Work?"

Contraception is arguably seen as "women's work;" hence the assumption that men will not use it. Indeed, the field of reproductive science and medicine has focused mainly on women's bodies, and has neglected men's.[6] Yet gender roles are changing, and today, men are more likely to share in household and childcare responsibilities. This rebalancing may extend to contraception, with studies suggesting that younger men are more likely to see it as a shared responsibility. Certain groups of men, particularly those who are more educated and affluent, and who place less importance on traditional gender roles, are more likely to be supportive of, and even eager for, male contraception.

One third of sexually active British men say they would consider using hormonal contraception, such as the pill or an implant. This is the same proportion of British women who currently use such medication. Eight out of 10 people in the survey said contraception should be a shared responsibility. Meanwhile, in a survey of sexually active men aged 18–44 in the United States, 77% said they are "very or somewhat" interested in trying out a male contraceptive other than condoms or vasectomy (Campo-Engelstein 2019). Thus, could public acceptance, alongside a relaxation of gender roles, lead to the male pill becoming a reality?

Sanger and McCormick made it clear, at the time, that they were not interested in a birth control pill for men. They did not trust men to take the responsibility, and they wanted women to possess control of their own bodies and their own fertility (Eig 2014). Surely, when the female pill was mass produced in the early 1960s,

---

[6] For instance, everyone knows what a gynecologist does, yet relatively few will have heard of an andrologist, a doctor who specializes in the male reproductive system.

women could control their fertility, for the first time, without their sexual partner's knowledge or involvement. Nevertheless, as society seems to be moving toward greater gender equality, some argue that it is striking how women remain the ones who must experience the emotional, social, financial, and time-related burdens of contraception, not to mention the side effects (Campo-Engelstein 2019).

Research on the male pill not only started decades after the female pill, but it has also been held back by lack of funding. This is partly because pharmaceutical companies, regulators, and men themselves appear less accepting of potential side effects. While certain symptoms are considered acceptable in female contraceptives, because they are weighed against the risks of pregnancy, they are often viewed as "deal breakers" for male contraceptives, because the comparison group is healthy young men. Additionally, common side effects of the female pill such as weight gain, mood swings, and lowered sex drive are often seen as emasculating. Research on the "clean sheets" pill, a male contraceptive that enables a semen-free orgasm, has stalled for similar reasons, because ejaculation is seen as an important component of male sexuality[16] (Campo-Engelstein 2019).

Nevertheless, it took only a decade for the female pill to be made widely available after it was invented. So why is it taking so long to market the male pill, which was first trialed in the 1970s? (Wang et al. 2016). Some scientists claim that the science of developing male contraceptives is more complicated than developing female contraceptives.[16] Yet already a decade ago, scientists claimed to have developed a male contraceptive that was 100% effective and side-effect free in trials.[19] Obviously, while welcome, the mass availability of a male pill will not ensure its usage—an issue seen also with sterilization rates. Male vasectomy was invented almost 200 years ago, but female sterilization is still 10 times more common worldwide, despite being less effective, more expensive, and more prone to complications. As Lisa Campo-Engelstein, from the Albany Medical School, rightly points out, greater gender equality is a necessary first step in removing social and economic barriers to developing male contraceptives: "we have been waiting 50 years for a male pill, let's not wait another 50." (Campo-Engelstein 2019).

5.8 Conclusions

After examining the history of the pill, I became aware of how lucky I was that it was available when I needed it. Today, however, young women—and those who are not so young—may be unaware of the enormous struggle that the pill's development involved. Indeed, at the start of the third decade of the twenty-first century, it is not easy to envisage the huge difficulties that faced Margaret Sanger, Katharine McCormick, Gregory Pincus, and John Rock when making the pill available for women worldwide—only 60 years ago.

The two "mothers" of the pill insisted that female control of contraception was a prerequisite for women's emancipation. Since women disproportionately bore the burden of pregnancy and child rearing, they believed that women should have a contraceptive controlled by them alone. Both women believed that birth control would help women overcome some of the fundamental inequalities of being women: that it would liberate them to seek more education, pursue better jobs, and raise healthier and better-educated children. To achieve their goal, they enlisted the help of the scientist Gregory Pincus who enrolled a Catholic physician, John Rock, in their struggle. In creating the pill, the two women activists ushered in what one historian called "the contraceptive mentality"—the belief in the right of a woman to control her own fertility. Family planning was the euphemism used by Sanger to make the idea of contraception more palatable to politicians and policy makers. Today, the WHO—but not only the WHO—uses both terms interchangeably and promotes contraception and family planning worldwide.

It was certainly ironic that the great sexual revolution in the United States came as Sanger remade her crusade. A mission that had originally been built around the joy of sex and the desire for more was reconstructed around respectable themes such as population control and sound parenthood. But Sanger's dream had come true; as Americans now believe that sexuality need not be restricted by social conventions. Recent generations have a higher number of sexual partners as adults and have more casual sex than those born earlier in the twentieth century.

In the context of womb politics, through the decades, the pill has liberated many women, allowing them to either postpone or prevent motherhood in favor of other opportunities, such as higher education and employment. This is one reason why it is often viewed as a key milestone for women's rights, and one of the greatest inventions of the twentieth century. Indeed, in 1938, the Comstock laws were overturned and birth control is currently widely accepted and used on a par with family planning.

However, women's struggle in the abortion camp is a different story.

The next chapter explores abortion wars.

Notes

(1) https://www.plannedparenthood.org/planned-parenthood-massachusetts/who-we-are/our-history. Accessed 2 Jan 2020.
(2) http://news.bbc.co.uk/onthisday/hi/dates/stories/december/4/newsid_3228000/3228207.stm. Accessed 2 Jan 2020.
(3) https://www.pbs.org/wgbh/americanexperience/films/pill/. The Pill. Accessed 2 Mar 2020.
(4) https://www.britannica.com/biography/Margaret-Sanger. Accessed 2 Jan 2020.
(5) https://amazingwomeninhistory.com/katharine-mccormick-birth-control-history/. Accessed 2 Jan 2020.
(6) https://www.pbs.org/wgbh/americanexperience/features/pill-boston-pill-trials/. Accessed 2 Jan 2020.
(7) https://www.pbs.org/wgbh/americanexperience/features/pill-dr-john-rock-1890-1984/. Accessed 2 Jan 2020.

(8)   Encyclical Letter Humanae Vitae of the Supreme Pontiff Paul VI. http://www.vatican.
      va/content/paul-vi/en/encyclicals/documents/hf_p-vi_enc_25071968_humanae-vitae.html.
      Accessed 2 Jan 2021.
(9)   https://www.pbs.org/wgbh/americanexperience/features/pill-america/. Accessed 2 Jan 2020.
(10) https://news.bbc.co.uk/onthisday/hi/dates/stories/december/4/newsid_3228000/322820
      7/stm. Accessed 2 Jan 2020.
(11) https://www.pbs.org/wgbh/americanexperience/features/pill-and-womens-liberation-mov
      ement/. Accessed 2 Jan 2020.
(12) https://www.pbs.org/wgbh/americanexperience/films/pill/ThePill. Accessed 2 Mar 2020.
(13) https://www.pbs.org/wgbh/americanexperience/features/pill-senate-holds-hearings-pill-
      1970/. Accessed 3 Jan 2020.
(14) https://www.plannedparenthood.org/learn/birth-control/birth-control-pill. Accessed 2 Jan
      2020.
(15) Oral contraceptives and cancer risk. (2012, March 21) https://www.cancer.gov/about-cancer/
      causes-prevention/risk/hormones/oral-contraceptives-fact-sheet. Accessed 2 Aug 2021.
(16) https://www.pbs.org/wgbh/americanexperience/features/pill-current-pill-use/. Current Pill
      Use (Originally published in 2003).
(17) What is an IUD? https://www.medicalnewstoday.com/articles/314368.php#how-to-safely-
      switch.
(18) https://www.webmd.com/sex/birth-control/birth-control-pills#1. Accessed 2 Jan 2020.
(19) http://news.bbc.co.uk/1/hi/health/3167090.stm. Updated: Jul 28, 2019; Original: Feb 9, 2010.
      Accessed 2 Jan 2020.

References

Ambrosino, Brandon. 2019. *Are We Set for a New Sexual Revolution?* https://www.bbc.com/future/
      article/20190702-are-we-set-for-a-new-sexual-revolution. Accessed 3 Jan 2020.
Campo-Engelstein, Lisa. 2019. *Are We Ready for Men to Take the Pill? Albany Medical College.*
      https://www.bbc.co.uk/news/health-49879667. Accessed 2 Jan 2020.
Castelman, M. 2014, November 15. How Birth Control Pills Affect Women's Sexu-
      ality. *Psychology Today.* https://www.psychologytoday.com/blog/all-about-sex/201411/how-
      birth-control-pills-affect-womens-sexuality; https://www.cdc.gov/reproductivehealth/contracep
      tion/index.htm. Accessed 2 Jan 2020.
Eig, Jonathan. 2014. *The Birth of the Pill.* London: Macmillan.
Kirtane, Ameya R., Tiffany Hua, Alison Hayward, Ambika Bajpayee, Aniket Wahane, et al. 2019.
      A Once-A-Month Oral Contraceptive. *Science Translational Medicine* 2019 (11): 521. https://
      doi.org/10.1126/scitranslmed.aay2602
Lewis, Jone Johnson. 2019. *The History of the Comstock Law.* https://www.thoughtco.com/history-
      of-the-comstock-law-3529472. Accessed 2 Jan 2020.
Lopez, L.M., S. Ramesh, M. Chen, A. Edelman, C. Otterness, J. Trussell, and F.M. Helmerhorst.
      2016, August 28. Progestin-Only Contraceptives: Effects on Weight. *Cochrane Database of
      Systematic Reviews* 2016 (8) Art. No.: CD008815. https://www.ncbi.nlm.nih.gov/pubmedhealth/
      PMH0014869/. Accessed 3 Jan 2020.
Migraine and the Contraceptive Pill. n.d. https://www.migrainetrust.org/living-with-migraine/cop
      ing-managing/contraceptive-pill/. Accessed 2 Jan 2020.
Platoni, Kara. 2010. *The Sex Scholar. Stanford Magazine.* https://stanfordmag.org/contents/the-sex-
      scholar. Accessed 2 Mar 2020.

Smith, Lori. 2018. *Medically Reviewed by Debra Rose Wilson.* https://www.medicalnewstoday.com/articles/290196.php. Accessed 2 Mar 2020.

Tzankova, V., V. Petrov, and N. Danchev. 2010. Impact of Oral Contraceptives and Smoking on Arterial and Deep Venous Thrombosis: A Retrospective Case-Control Study. *Biotechnology & Biotechnological Equipment* 24 (3): 2026–2030. https://doi.org/10.2478/V10133-010-0054-Y.

Wang, Christina, Mario P. R. Festin, and Ronald S. Swerdloff. 2016. Male Hormonal Contraception: Where Are We Now? *Current Obstetrics and Gynecology Reports* 5: 38–47.

WHO. 2018. *Family Planning/Contraception.* 8 February 2018. https://www.who.int/news-room/fact-sheets/detail/family-planning-contraception. Accessed 5 Jan 2020.

Chapter 6
The Abortion Wars

We know that the male colonization of mothers' bodies starts inside the womb. (Jacqueline Rose 2019, p. 54)

Conceiving a child is widely considered a happy event. The advent of IVF has highlighted the joy of this common occurrence, by loudly and publicly disclosing the misery and despair of couples who wish to have a child but are incapable of conceiving (see also Chap. 6). Stories, in the twentieth century, of desperate women who were unable to conceive have enhanced many of the current idealizations and romanticisms about pregnancy and childbirth in addition to the first biblical mandate: "Be fertile and replenish the earth" (see Chap. 2). Religious belief and romantic views can make a pregnancy bearable.

Romanticism aside, from a pure biologic perspective, the fetus is a parasite that takes over a woman's body and grows at her expense (see also Chap. 9).[1] If the pregnancy is desired and expected, though, a woman may be genuinely happy to bear the fetus for nine months to give birth to a wanted baby. In the case of unwanted pregnancy, a woman has the option to either abort the fetus or to continue with the pregnancy nevertheless. If the second option is chosen, the newborn, although not planned, may become a wanted child. But if the feeling of an unwelcome pregnancy persists, the result is an unwanted child. Childhood is not easy; but being unwanted can mean a hellish life for a child—and for the mother. This chapter explores elective termination of pregnancy. It looks at the incidence of abortions worldwide, examines the legality of the procedure and the situation of abortion in the United States (as an example of a country in which abortion is legal) and in Israel (where abortion is illegal).

---

[1] For example, I fainted a few hours after giving birth to my daughter, because my hemoglobin (Hb) was 7.5 g/d (grams per deciliter) while the lower norm is Hb 11 g/d. And no, I did not have a bad hemorrhage during delivery. In contrast, my baby daughter had a perfect count of Hb 13 g/d. During her stay in my womb, she had efficiently taken from me all the iron she needed to build her own hemoglobin. This is exactly what a fetus does while in the womb.

This chapter deals only with induced abortions.

© The Author(s), under exclusive license to Springer Nature Switzerland AG 2022
F. Simonstein, *Womb Politics: A Short History of the Future of Human Reproduction*,
The International Library of Bioethics 99,
https://doi.org/10.1007/978-3-031-11654-4_5

6.1   Abortion

A Woman's Right Over Her Body?

If the pregnancy is not desired, the woman in question can experience conceiving as an appalling and frightening event; the sensation is of being trapped in your own body. This was my experience. I was 23 years old, already the happy mother of two wanted children, a girl and a boy (aged 6 years and 2 years, respectively). Since I had decided not to have more children, I was on the pill; but I got pregnant. I decided to terminate this pregnancy, and was lucky enough to have the abortion safely at a private clinic.[2] Six months later, I became pregnant again. I decided to terminate that pregnancy, as well (after which I asked for an IUD). My two abortions were tough, both physically and mentally, but I understood that, for me, the alternative would be much worse. Nevertheless, on both occasions, the nurse on the kibbutz in Israel, where I lived at the time, tried to persuade me not to terminate the pregnancies, insisting that I would regret it later. I have never regretted it. For me, it was the right decision and I am writing about it openly in this book. Although women who have had abortions do not generally chat about the subject, over the years I discovered that many women around me—including my mother, my mother-in-law, two aunts, and two younger women in the family—went through this procedure at some point. These abortions took place in three different countries, in two of them clandestinely. Clearly, more women than we may think have abortions, either overtly or covertly.

I was lucky to get through the abortions in the 1970s. It was illegal then—as I found out many years later—but you could find a good physician who would perform the procedure safely in his clinic. Nowadays, the law prohibiting abortions in Israel has become more stringent. Physicians would not proceed with an abortion without its legalization, even in a private setting, and Israel is not the only country where this is the case. Currently, in the second decade of the twenty-first century, women, worldwide, who do not wish to continue with a pregnancy, cannot terminate it if they so desire.

Such a state of affairs is a loud and clear manifestation of the politics of the womb. A woman who does not wish to continue a pregnancy must ask the permission of the state to have an abortion. If she is lucky, living in a country that permits "abortion, but...," and she fulfills the requirements imposed on her by the state (the reason/s for the abortion, the week of the pregnancy), she might be allowed a termination.

---

[2] During the two years prior to this pregnancy, my daughter had been hospitalized three times, for a full month each time. She had a blood condition (Recurrent Thrombocytopenia Purpura, R-TPP), which luckily disappeared before puberty. During those two years, my son was hospitalized twice as well—when he was just 6 weeks old for an urgent operation (Hernia Incarcerata)—and again at 10 months because of severe diarrhea (due to ear infection). Luckily, in my son's case, these conditions were quickly resolved, but my daughter's illness, R-TTP, reappeared again and again— intermittently—for the next 6 years. Throughout those difficult years, I became well aware of how taxing and difficult child rearing can be, and of the responsibilities inherent to parenting—even without sickness and hospitalizations—for a lifetime.

Otherwise, she is forced to continue until the birth. In short, in most parts of the world, a woman cannot decide what to do with her own body.

6.2 Abortion Worldwide

According to the Guttmacher Institute's executive summary in 2017, the vast majority of abortions are the result of unintended pregnancies. Globally, 56% of unintended pregnancies end in induced abortion; regionally, this proportion ranges from 36% in North America to 70% in Europe.[1] According to a report by the World Health Organization (WHO) in 2019, an average of 56 million induced abortions (safe and unsafe) per year took place worldwide from 2010–2014.[2] This corresponds to approximately 125,000 abortions per day. On the Worldometer website, by mid-February 2020, the abortion count had already reached almost 6 million.[3] From 2010 to 2014, an estimated 36 abortions were performed each year per 1000 women aged 15–44 in developing regions, compared with 27 abortions in developed regions. There was a decline in abortion rates in Eastern Europe and in the developing sub-region of Central Asia, where use of effective contraceptives increased dramatically. Both sub-regions are made up of former Soviet Bloc states where the availability of modern contraceptives increased sharply after political independence—exemplifying how the abortion rate decreases with elevated use of effective contraceptives.[1]

Of all abortions, an estimated 55% are *safe* (i.e., performed using a recommended method and by an appropriately trained provider); 31% are *less safe* (i.e., meet either method or provider criterion), and 14% are *least safe* (meet neither criterion). The more restrictive the legal setting, the higher the percentage of least-safe abortions—ranging from less than 1% in the least-restrictive countries to 31% in the most-restrictive countries. In addition, persistent stigma can affect the willingness of providers to offer abortions and may lead women to prioritize secrecy over safety. Most importantly, abortions occur as frequently in the two most-restrictive categories of countries (banned outright or allowed only to save the woman's life) as in the least-restrictive category (allowed without restriction as to reason)—37 and 34 per 1000 women, respectively. Thus, highly restrictive laws do not eliminate the practice of abortion, but raise the likelihood that those that do occur will be unsafe.[1]

According to Jonathan Eig (2014), wanting to terminate a pregnancy is not a novelty. As seen in the previous chapter, the methods used to end a pregnancy, up to the advent of the contraception pill were harsh, highly dangerous, and ineffective. Human rights bodies have repeatedly condemned restrictive abortion laws as being incompatible with human rights norms.[4] Other institutions, however, continue to fight against abortion rights. Disturbingly, a book published recently, and its website, for example, claim that abortion has been "the greatest genocide" perpetrated on earth (2018). As a result of antiabortion policies worldwide—in the third decade of the twenty-first century—women are still not at liberty to terminate a pregnancy. Either abortion is illegal, or, if it is legal, the country's abortion legislation includes restrictions. Thus, even if abortion in the country is legal, a woman is required to ask permission from the state—that comprises mostly men—to terminate a pregnancy. And she may not get that permission.[3]

6.3 [I]Legal Abortion

According to the WHO, in most countries, women do not have access to safe abortion care: abortion is legal in only 28% of all countries in the world and only 15% of countries in the developing world. Laws fall along a continuum from outright prohibition to allowing abortion without restriction as to reason (World Health Organization 2011). Many women who live in countries where abortion is legally available are unable to access a safe procedure, for many reasons, including a lack of knowledge about the legal status of abortion, lack of money to pay for the procedure, social stigma against abortion or, commonly, because they present for care too far along in pregnancy.[5]

According to 2017 data, 42% of women of reproductive age live in the 125 countries where abortion is highly restricted (prohibited altogether, or allowed only to save a woman's life or protect her health)[6] (World Health Organization 2011; Johnson et al. 2018). Nine hundred and seventy million women, representing 58% of women of reproductive age, live in countries that broadly allow abortion. Whereas the majority of women live in countries where they can exercise their right to abortion, 42% live under restrictive laws. The inability to access safe and legal abortion care impacts 700 million women of reproductive age. Moreover, legal restrictions on abortion do not result in fewer abortions; instead, they compel women to risk their lives and health by seeking out unsafe abortion care.[4] According to recent estimates, at least 8% of maternal deaths worldwide are from unsafe abortion; 23,000 women die of unsafe abortion each year and tens of thousands more experience significant health complications.[4],[7]

The lawfulness of abortion—i.e., the allowed or permitted categories of abortion as expressed through laws, policies, and guidelines—is a key component of a facilitating environment for safe abortion. The continuum of lawful abortion ranges from abortion at a woman's request with no requirement for justification, through specified grounds, uncertain prohibition where laws prohibit unlawful abortion but do not specify any lawful grounds, to prohibition of all abortions. It is noteworthy, however, that where abortion is lawful, access can be restricted by gestational age, requirements for third-party authorizations, and an assortment of service-delivery requirements[8] (Johnson et al. 2018).

Categories of Abortion Laws

The categories of lawful abortion, and how they are expressed in law and policy, have implications for who decides whether a woman is eligible, as well as when,

---

[3] Moreover, the development of new technologies (AWs) that support earlier viability of newborns (fetuses, in fact) may impose further challenges to abortion schemes (see Chap. 8).

where, and by whom abortion services can be provided[4],[9] (Johnson et al. 2018). The following categories are based on the interactive map center for reproductive rights.[4]

Category 1
Prohibited Altogether. The laws of the countries in this category do not permit abortion under any circumstances, including when the woman's life or health are at risk. Globally, 26 countries fall within this category, and **90 million** women of reproductive age (5%) live in countries that prohibit abortion altogether.

Category II
To Save a Woman's Life. The laws of the countries in this category permit abortion when the woman's life is at risk. The 39 countries in this category include **359 million** women of reproductive age (22%) who are resident in these countries.

Category III
To Preserve Health. The laws of countries in this category permit abortion on health or therapeutic grounds. Resident in these countries are **237 million** women of reproductive age (14%).

Category IV
Broad Social or Economic Grounds. These laws are generally interpreted liberally to permit abortion under a broad range of circumstances. These countries often consider a woman's actual or reasonably foreseeable environment and her social or economic circumstances when considering the potential impact of pregnancy and childbearing (United Kindom and Finland here). This category includes **386 million** women of reproductive age (23%) living in countries that allow abortion on broad social or economic grounds.

Category V
On Request (gestational limits vary): four countries.

No indications stated: eight countries (mostly from the former Soviet Union, including Russia).

Out of 163 countries on earth, only eight have no indication for abortion (mostly from the former Soviet Union, including Russia).[9] Restrictions are in place in 102 countries and 61 countries have "no restrictions." However, in some countries in which abortion is permitted, the limitations are at least as restrictive, and even more so, than in countries where abortion is illegal. Thus, in 92% of all countries, women must get permission to terminate a pregnancy.[9] Around 600 million women (36%) live where abortion is allowed without restriction as to reason. Almost 100 million women of reproductive age (6%) live where abortion is banned. And the remaining women, close to 1 billion, live in countries with laws that fall between these two extremes.[7] This means that more than 1 billion women (64%) live in countries that have abortion restrictions.

Although the Guttmacher Institute tries to project some optimism by writing that the situation is improving somewhat, the overall numbers remain appalling. What is more, the United States is counted among the three "no restriction" countries, together with Puerto Rico and the Netherlands. However, while the US is regarded as a developed country where abortion was made legal, many restrictions are in place and mounting. Only some U.S. states do not have a gestational limit for pre-viability abortion. Furthermore, the legality of abortion in the United States is continuously under threat. The next section focuses on the legality of abortion there.

6.4   Abortion in the United States

The United States is counted among the countries in which abortion is legal. However, restrictions by state are permitted—and mounting. Since the Supreme Court handed down its Roe v. Wade decision in 1973, legalizing abortion in the US, different states have constructed a complicated abortion law, codifying, regulating and limiting whether, when, and under which circumstances a woman may obtain an abortion. The following points highlight the major provisions of these state laws.[10]

- Seventeen states require the involvement of a second physician after a specified point. In 33 states and the District of Columbia, the use of state funds is prohibited, except in those cases when federal funds are available: when the woman's life is in danger or when the pregnancy is the result of rape or incest. In defiance of federal requirements, South Dakota limits funding to cases of life endangerment only.
- *Gestational Limits*: In 43 states, abortions are prohibited, generally, except when necessary to protect the woman's life or health, after a specified point in pregnancy.
- *Refusal:* In 45 states, individual health care providers are entitled to refuse to participate in an abortion. In 42 states, institutions are allowed to refuse to perform abortions. In 16 of these states, refusal is limited to private or religious institutions.
- *State-Mandated Counseling*: Eighteen states mandate that, before an abortion, women be given counseling that includes information on at least one of the following: the purported link between abortion and breast cancer (5 states), the ability of a fetus to feel pain (13 states), or long-term mental health consequences for the woman (8 states).
- *Waiting Periods*: In 27 states, a woman seeking an abortion is required to wait a specified period, usually 24 h, between receiving counseling and performance of the procedure. Fourteen of these states have laws that effectively require the woman to make two separate trips to the clinic to obtain the procedure.
- *Parental Involvement*: In 37 states, some type of parental involvement is required in a minor's decision to have an abortion.

Republican legislators have successfully pushed through abortion restriction bills by targeting providers, for example through mandating waiting periods for patients or offering privileges to hospital doctors who refuse to perform abortions (personal communication). Many states limited the procedure to 22 weeks, but until 2019, 6-week bans were largely seen as too extreme; two that passed, in Iowa and North Dakota, were later struck down in court. Abortion rights advocates say limiting the procedure to earlier than 6 weeks into the pregnancy is effectively a complete ban, since most women do not learn that they are pregnant until later[11] (Gay 2014). Nevertheless, in May 2019, the legislature of Missouri passed a ban on abortions, among the most extreme of any state. The ban prohibits any abortions after 8 weeks of gestation, putting it in the category of misleadingly named "heartbeat bills" that use fetal cardiac activity as a marker, in fact, for illegality. Like a law signed in 2019 in Alabama, the Missouri bill contains no exceptions for cases of rape or incest (Rogers 2019).

In 2019, limits on abortion changed also in the states of Georgia, Kentucky, Louisiana, Missouri, Mississippi, and Ohio, which stopped short of outright bans, instead passing so-called heartbeat bills that effectively prohibit abortions after 6 to 8 weeks of pregnancy, when doctors can usually start detecting a fetal heartbeat.That makes eight U.S. states, with similar extreme bans on their books, each vying to be the law that makes its way to the Supreme Court, and overturns Roe v. Wade, the 1973 decision that legalized abortion in the United States.[11] The next section explores Roe v. Wade—a landmark case in the US.

Roe v. Wade

Texas law made it a felony to abort a fetus except "on medical advice for the purpose of saving the life of the mother." Texas resident Jane Roe was unmarried and pregnant in 1970. Roe filed a suit against Wade, the district attorney of Dallas County, contesting the statute on the grounds that it violated the guarantee of personal liberty and the right to privacy implicitly guaranteed in the First, Fourth, Fifth, Ninth, and Fourteenth Amendments.[12] Previously, on June 7, 1965, in Griswold v. State of Connecticut, the U.S. Supreme Court had decided in favor of the constitutional right of married persons to use birth control. This privacy case was also cited in *Roe* v. *Wade*.[13] In deciding for Roe, the Supreme Court invalidated any state laws that prohibited first trimester abortions.The written opinion for the majority recognized that a woman's choice of whether or not to have an abortion is protected by her right to privacy. Two justices dissented, however. The majority determined that a woman's right to decide whether to have an abortion involved the question of whether the Constitution protected *a right to privacy*. The justices answered this question by asserting that the Fourteenth Amendment, which prohibits states from "depriv[ing] any person of … liberty … without due process of law," protected a fundamental right to privacy. Furthermore, after discussing the law's historical lack of recognition of rights of a fetus, the justices concluded that "the word 'person,' as used in the 14th Amendment, does not include the unborn." The right of a woman to choose to have an abortion fell within this fundamental right to privacy and was protected by the Constitution.[12] Nonetheless, it is important to note that even in this landmark case that permitted abortion in the United States, a woman's right to choose to have an abortion was *not* considered an absolute right. Why? We may find the answer in the following statement:

We ... acknowledge our awareness of the sensitive and emotional nature of the abortion controversy, of the vigorous opposing views, even among physicians, and of the deep and seemingly absolute convictions that the subject inspires—Justice Blackmun (1973), majority opinion in Roe v. Wade.[12]

Thus, the majority of the justices in Roe v. Wade regarded the opposition to abortion as something "respectable." Moreover, although the majority of the justices in this trial accepted that a woman's choice as to whether or not to have an abortion is protected by her right to privacy, they also added that "states did have some 'legitimate interests' in regulating or prohibiting abortions."[12]

According to Roe v. Wade, the first interest of the state is the protection of the health of the mother from "the dangers of abortion procedures" (I will return to this in a moment); the second interest is the protection of the life of the fetus. While these interests, in their opinion, are not very strong in the early stages of pregnancy, they become stronger (more compelling) in the later stages. Striking a balance between a woman's right to privacy and a state's interests, the Court set up a framework laying down when states could regulate and even prohibit abortions as follows:

...in the first trimester (the first three months of the pregnancy), a woman's right to privacy surrounding the choice to have an abortion outweighed a state's interests in regulating this decision. In the first trimester, having an abortion does not pose a grave danger to the life and health of the mother, and the fetus is still undeveloped. The state's interests are *not yet compelling*, so it cannot interfere with a woman's right to privacy by regulating or prohibiting her from having an abortion during the first trimester. During the second trimester, the state's interests become more compelling as the danger of complications increases and the fetus becomes more developed. During this stage, it may regulate, but not prohibit abortions, as long as the regulations are aimed at protecting the health of the mother. During the third trimester, the danger to the woman's health becomes the greatest and fetal development nears completion. In the final trimester *the state's interests* in protecting the health of the mother and in protecting the life of the fetus become their most compelling. The state may regulate or even prohibit abortions during this stage, as long as there is an exception for abortions necessary to preserve the life and health of the mother [my italics].[12]

Furthermore, in his dissenting opinion, one of the judges argued that this issue—abortion—requires "a careful balance of the interests of the woman against the interests of the state;" so it was not an appropriate decision for the Court to make, but instead was "a question that should have been left up to state legislatures to resolve."[12] While this was a dissenting opinion against making abortion legal, the framework legalizing abortion itself includes three instances of the words "state interests." This means that the interest of the state may overrule a woman's desire to terminate a pregnancy. It is no wonder, then, that some states have taken to expanding their "state interests;" and as the following case demonstrates, have tried to overrule Roe.

Planned Parenthood of Southeastern Pennsylvania et al. v. Robert P. Casey et al.

This was a significant case in terms of abortion laws. It was the first case since *Roe v. Wade* to attempt to change abortion laws and was settled in 1992.[14] The case revolved around the issue of consent in abortions, for example, a woman's obligation to wait 24 h before having the procedure. The Pennsylvania Abortion Control Act of 1982 contained five controversial provisions:

1. Doctors were required to inform women considering abortion about its potential negative impacts on their health.
2. Women were required to give notice to husbands before obtaining an abortion.
3. Children were required to get consent from a parent or guardian.
4. A 24-h waiting period was required between deciding to have an abortion and undergoing the procedure.
5. Reporting requirements were imposed on facilities offering abortions.[14]

Many of the Pennsylvania restrictions on abortion law were considered unconstitutional, and the case arrived at the Supreme Court. The plaintiffs, comprising several abortion clinics and abortion-providing doctors, argued that the Pennsylvania restrictions on abortion were unconstitutional and violated a woman's rights. On the other side, this was viewed as an opportunity to challenge the right of abortion provided by Roe v. Wade as the Court was now more conservative. Republican President George W.H. Bush had appointed two new Justices considered to be less liberal than the two retired Democratic appointees. There were now eight Republican appointees and only two Justices who had previously shown support for Roe. This court could overturn Roe v. Wade. Thus, the odds were against the pro-choice advocates from the start.

Nonetheless, the plurality in the U.S. Court of Appeals rejected the call to overturn Roe v. Wade (which the state had advanced on appeal) and reaffirmed the existence of a constitutional right to abortion. However, although the decision maintained *Roe v. Wade*, many of the provisions in the Pennsylvania law were upheld, in a very close 5–4 battle. The plurality struck down only the spousal notice requirement but upheld the remaining contested regulations—the State's informed consent and 24-h waiting period, parental consent requirements, reporting requirements, and the "medical emergencies" definition—holding that none constituted an undue burden.[14]

Moreover, while Roe v. Wade survived, the U.S. Court of Appeals reshaped against some of Roe's guidelines. The plurality found that a fetus could become viable earlier than when Roe was decided and held that a state could ban abortion once a fetus becomes viable unless the health of the mother is at risk. Its other revision of Roe was its replacement of "strict scrutiny" with an "undue burden standard that was more lenient to the state."[15]

In addition, the Court was deeply divided on this case. For instance, two Justices would have upheld all of the provisions, including the spousal notification requirement, and thought also that the Court should have used this opportunity to overrule Roe entirely. Four Justices upheld that:

...a woman's decision to abort her unborn child is not a constitutionally protected "liberty" because (1) the Constitution says absolutely nothing about it, and (2) *the long-standing traditions of American society* have permitted it to be legally proscribed. 841(7) [my italics].[16]

To sum up, this case upheld that states may regulate abortion procedures in ways related to "a legitimate state interest;" clearly against a woman's right over her own body. Obviously the door remained open for future challenges to Roe.[4]

Most importantly, in both Roe and Casey cases, the "state interest" is quoted over the womb. Thus, the state has a "legitimate" claim over a woman's body. The following section includes three different cases of "state's interest" on abortion, in which "the state" has also become the owner of women's bodies. For example, the interest of the state in deciding what a woman should and should not do with her own body was at the center of the Romanian case.[5]

6.5   The State's Interest in Abortion

The Interest of the State I: Romanian Case

The Romanian case is one of the well-known—and horrific—examples of where the "interests of the state" may lead desperate women when the law dictates that they bring their pregnancies to term. Abortion was legal in Romania until 1966, when Nicolai Ceausescu became President and outlawed it, along with contraception. The rationale behind this was his aim to increase the number of native-born Romanians. Women were forced to have pelvic inspections at work! Police informers roamed maternity hospitals. Performing abortions was a crime. As a result, the birth rate in Romania went up for a couple years, and then in 1970, went into freefall. Deaths from complications resulting from attempted illegal abortions increased to 10 times that of the rest of Europe—about 500 women a year, more than 10,000 women over two decades. The maternal mortality rate spiked to 150 women per 100,000 births, which is an insanely high number. Today, when the United States has the worst maternal mortality in the industrialized world, it is only a sixth of that (except in Louisiana, where the maternal mortality rate for women over 35 years of age is a 1980s-Romania-adjacent 145.9 per 100,000 births). In addition, nearly 200,000 children were placed in hellish orphanages (Rogers 2019).

In December1989, a revolution cleared out Ceausescu's government. The new leadership instituted an emergency public health measure to legalize abortion and contraception. The maternal mortality rate fell by 50% in the first year. In Romania, abortion mortality skyrocketed because people were doing things illegally. Indeed, when abortion is illegal, it can be extremely unsafe. The Romanian case clearly exposes what happens when the interests of the state appropriate women's bodies at the expense of and irrespective of women's wishes (Rogers 2019). It is an extreme example of how the interest of the state has exerted power over women's bodies. Yet

---

[4] On May 2002 a leaked draft by the Supreme Court appeared, aiming to abolish Roe (according to the press).

[5] By "state" here, I do not refer to the American framework but to the political directive of a country.

the interest of the state is also reflected in other—less horrendous—cases of women being subjected to abortion restrictions.

The Interest of the State II: Abortion in Israel

The termination of my unwanted pregnancies took place in the 1970s in Israel, where abortion is illegal. At that time, I could have an abortion privately with no further questions asked. I was unaware that the procedure was illegal. Since then, however, the abortion law in Israel has been reinforced. A woman who wishes to terminate a pregnancy in Israel must appeal to a committee of three people (two physicians and a person representing "the public," usually a social worker). In Israel today, a gynecologist would not perform an abortion, even privately, without approval signed by the authorization committee.

The Israeli law permits abortion under six conditions: if the pregnancy results from rape; if the woman is under 18 or over 45; if the fetus carries a genetic disease; if the pregnancy threatens the woman's life, and if the pregnancy is the result of adultery. If the reason for the abortion appeal coincides with any of these cases, the committee would authorize a woman to terminate her pregnancy. Under any other circumstances, she would not be allowed to abort. Thus, in Israel as well, a woman must request authorization by "the state" to determine what happens to her own body. For it is in "the interest of the state" that women in Israel do not terminate a pregnancy. Under the present law, Israeli women must continue to carry the fetus and give birth, irrespective of their wishes. So, if women do not want to continue with the pregnancy for any other reason—such as alternative life plans or the inability to care for more children—what do they do? It is noteworthy that the rate of legal abortions in Israel is high (Kamin 2014; Sharon 2019). In 2018, for example, out of the 17,869 women who applied to have an abortion, 99.2% received the committee's approval. According to Israel's Central Bureau of Statistics, the most frequent motive (50.9%) for all the abortions authorized by the termination committee in 2019 was that the pregnancy occurred outside wedlock.[17]

It would seem, then, that Israeli married women are particularly promiscuous. But the truth is that if the woman wants to terminate her pregnancy—for any reason other than those permitted by law—her gynecologist would counsel her to tell the committee that the child is not her husband's, making a legal case for abortion (personal communication). This might not be bad advice if we take a woman's options into account: either to continue with an unwanted pregnancy and deliver a child she does not want, or lying to the committee about the identity of the father.[6] According to the statistics, most women seem to choose the second option, but this may put the woman in a delicate position; husbands have already used such testimonies of illegitimacy to obtain an advantageous deal in a disputed divorce.[18] According to Jewish law, if the husband can prove adultery, the rabbinical court may order her

---

[6] Most women in Israel are granted the desired abortion. However, the fact that Israeli women untruthfully tell the committee that the child is not their husband's in order to obtain the authorization (making it "easier" to get) does not make abortion in Israel less illegal.

to divorce her husband on that basis.[7] In fact, Jewish law *requires* divorce when the wife commits a sexual transgression; the man must divorce her, even if he is inclined to forgive her.[(19)],[8] Thus, it appears that (almost) all women in Israel who apply for abortions obtain them legally. This is probably untrue, however, since according to the CBS, half of all women who receive the approval claim that the child is not their husband's. A declaration of adultery makes women vulnerable, because later, it may become a very useful weapon against her.[9]

The Interest of the State III: The Global Gag Rule

During summer 2005, I was a Senior WHO Research Fellow in the Department of Genetics. Wishing to understand the WHO's position on the situation of women in the area of genetic testing, I contacted the Women's Health Department. I was amazed to hear from a member of the department staff that any text from the Women's Health department containing the word "abortion" would be returned to the writer by Headquarters for rephrasing (personal communication). Why? The answer is very simple: the WHO's main source of funding at that time was U.S. President George W. Bush, so the word "abortion" was taboo. This was the interest of the state, according to the President of the United States.

The WHO's position clearly disregarded the fact that abortion is a part of women's reality worldwide. From 2010 to 2014, for example, 25% of all pregnancies ended in an induced abortion. During those years, 56 million (safe and unsafe) induced abortions occurred each year, on average, around the world.[(20)] If this is the case, how can one say that abortion is not relevant to women's health? The sad answer is that, in 2005, the WHO could not direct its health targets toward women's *real* needs. With the United States as its largest contributor—and with a Republican U.S. President who objected to abortion—the Global Gag Rule (GGR) was in place.

The Global Gag Rule (GGR)

The GGR prohibits foreign nongovernmental organizations (NGOs) who receive U.S. global health assistance from providing legal abortion services or referrals, while also barring advocacy for abortion law reform—even if the NGO uses its own

---

[7] Under Jewish law, a man can divorce a woman for any reason or no reason. The Talmud specifically says that a man can divorce a woman because she spoiled his dinner or simply because he finds another woman more attractive, and the woman's consent to the divorce is not required. http://www.jewfaq.org/divorce.htm

[8] In September 2006, the Great Rabbinical Court upheld a costs order made against an adulterous wife by Netanya Rabbinical Court. She had been ordered to pay her husband's legal fees in proving her adultery and his entitlement to divorce, as well as paying for the cost of the private detective he hired to produce the necessary evidence. http://www.family-laws.co.il/divorce-jewish-couples-mens-tactics.

[9] Presently, a Health Minister from a left-wing party in the Israeli government has announced plans to push legislative reforms that would return much of the decision-making power to women. However, in a wide but right-wing majority government (and the Knesset, including Orthodox Jewish parties), it is unlikely that these plans could be successful.

funds, unrelated to the US.[10] This policy allows access to abortion only in cases of rape, incest, or when a woman's life is at risk.[21] The GGR has been widely described as a "death warrant" for thousands of women[21] (Rose 2019; Ramaswamy 2019). Yet, Donald Trump reinstated the GGR on his first official day in office. According to Chitra Ramaswamy (among others), this was a "hateful rollback of women's right." Ramaswamy:

> The GGR represents a war on women: on their choices, lives, and on their internal organs. It is hard to think of a more unassailable right than the possession of one's own body. Of one's own womb. (Ramaswamy 2019, p. 163)

In January 2022, President Joseph Biden rescinded the GGR.[22] However, when the Republicans regain power, they will most probably reinstate it. The GGR puts thousands of doctors, midwives, and nurses all over the world in the unthinkable position of having to choose between offering family planning care—that includes abortion—and losing critical funding. Women die as a result, as unsafe abortions kill tens of thousands of women every single year[20] (Ramaswamy 2019). According to another WHO report in 2019, each year, between 4.7 and 13.2% of maternal deaths can be attributed to unsafe abortion. Around 7 million women are admitted to hospitals every year as a result of unsafe abortion (mostly in developing countries).[20] Unsafe abortion does serious damage to women. But some believe that safe abortion harms women as well.[5]

6.6   Does Abortion Do Damage to Women?

According to Roe v. Wade, one of the "legitimate interests of the state" is "the protection of the health of the mother from the dangers of abortion procedures."[12] This sounds very sensitive toward women. Nevertheless, it is an interesting way of caring, since the dangers involved in pregnancy and childbirth are far greater. The risk associated with a continued pregnancy is high, as 75% of global maternal deaths are a result of direct obstetric causes; and mortality associated with childbirth is approximately 14 times higher than that of abortion (Lavelanet et al. 2018).

In the mid-2000s, however, billboards worrying about the mental health of women who had had abortions were common, and justices in the Supreme Court expressed concern that those women might experience psychologically damaging "regret."[23] Was this actually true? Diana Greene Foster, a demographer and director of research at the Advancing New Standards in Reproductive Health program at the University of California, San Francisco, realized that most research looking at abortion outcomes compared women who had had an abortion to women who had become pregnant and had a baby.[24] This means that, in that research, the control group did not actually

---

[10] After this meeting, I understood why the Genetic Division at the WHO was soon to be terminated: the development of fetal genetic testing aimed at discovering if the fetus carries a genetic disease. Most probably, if the test would find that the fetus carries a dreadful genetic disease, parents would wish to terminate the pregnancy. Thus, against the GGR, an abortion would take place.

serve its purpose because it did not isolate the variable (Rogers 2019). What was really needed was a comparison between women with unwanted pregnancies who sought an abortion, and had one, with those who sought an abortion and were denied one. For abortion restrictions will certainly affect people who want abortions but who give birth, nonetheless. Thus, research should have looked at the effect on women who are able to have the desired abortion compared with the effect on women who were not.

The Turnaway Study

The Turnaway Study was a prospective longitudinal study examining the effects of unintended pregnancy on women's lives. The major aim of the study was to describe the mental health, physical health, and socioeconomic consequences of having an abortion compared to carrying an unwanted pregnancy to term.[5] From 2008 to 2010, approximately 1000 women who sought abortions were recruited from 30 abortion facilities around the United States; some who received abortions because they presented for care under the gestational limit of the clinic and some who were "turned away" and then carried to term because they were past the gestational limit.[24]

According to the findings of this study, abortion does not harm women. Abortion does not increase women's risk of having suicidal thoughts or the chance of developing PTSD, depression, anxiety, low self-esteem, or lower life satisfaction. Abortion does not increase women's use of alcohol, tobacco or drugs.[24] Yet women in the turnaway group were more likely to be poor 6 months after their visit to the clinic—and still to be poor 4 years later. Of the turnaways, those who continued to have children after their denied abortion had worse maternal bonding with their subsequent children than women who received an abortion and then had a child later. If a turnaway woman already had children—as 61% did—those children scored lower on standard measures of development, and were more likely to live below the federal poverty line in the years that followed. Half of these women gave the inability to afford to have a child as the reason for seeking an abortion.[25] Most importantly, the Turnaway Study found that women were confident about their decision to have an abortion, with 95% saying that abortion was the right decision for them. Moreover, women who received a wanted abortion were more likely to have a positive outlook on the future and achieve aspirational life plans within one year. As for the gestational limit, most women who sought abortion after 20 weeks had delayed because they did not know they were pregnant.[24]

My personal experience echoes the findings of this study: I never regretted terminating my unplanned pregnancies. This allowed me to go to university, to finish my first and second degrees, to get my PhD, and pursue an academic career.

6.7   Conclusions

Conceiving a child may be a happy event. However, if the pregnancy is not desired, the woman in question can experience conceiving as a terrible and frightening event.

The sensation for many women is of being trapped inside their bodies. And although most women who have undergone induced abortion do not generally chat about the subject, approximately 56 million induced abortions take place worldwide each year.

In addition to the physical and mental ordeal of abortion, women, almost everywhere, are not allowed to decide for themselves what to do with their own bodies. In more than 92% of all countries, women must get permission from the state to abort legally. Globally, either abortion is illegal altogether, illegal but permitted in some cases, or legal—in some countries. However, even if abortion is permitted, access can be restricted in that country by gestational age, requirements for third-party authorizations, and an assortment of service-delivery requirements. The development of new technologies (AWs) that support earlier viability of newborns (fetuses, in fact) may impose further challenges to abortion schemes (see Chap. 8).

Famously, the United States is included among the countries where abortion is legal. Roe v. Wade legalized abortion under the right of privacy. However, even in Roe v. Wade, "the interest of the state" may overrule the interest of the woman to end the pregnancy. States could regulate and even prohibit abortions, balancing between a woman's right to privacy and the state's interests. Thus, even in Roe v. Wade, the state remains the owner of women's bodies. Moreover, as mentioned above, the GGR prohibits foreign nongovernmental organizations (NGOs) who receive U.S. global health assistance from providing legal abortion services or referrals, while also barring advocacy for abortion law reform—even when using the NGO's own funds, independent of the US. And although in January 2022 Biden cancelled the GGR, most probably, when the Republicans return to power, they will re-establish it.

In any case, abortions occur as frequently in the two most-restrictive categories of countries as in the least-restrictive category. Thus, highly restrictive laws do not eliminate the practice of abortion, but make those that do occur more likely to be unsafe. Moreover, safe abortion does not harm women, and most women remain confident in their decision to terminate a pregnancy. According to the Guttmacher Institute, the situation may be improving, as some countries may now have expanded the categories in which abortion is allowed. However, it also recommends extending the legal grounds for abortion to give more women access to safer abortions. Indeed, around 1 billion women still have to obtain permission from the state—almost everywhere—to have an abortion.

Yet in the context of this book, the main and very basic question remains: if the pregnancy is unwanted, why on earth should a woman need to ask permission—from the state—to terminate it? On the other hand, help for women to become pregnant in the first place has been welcomed, celebrated, and copiously funded. So much so that, in Israel, women applying to the different commissions to receive IVF and to get a legal abortion find themselves in the same waiting room, one line in front of the other (personal communication). This "innocent" alignment may exacerbate the uncomfortable feelings that may be experienced by women seeking abortion in the first place. The message is clear: Look at the women in front of you, who desperately want a pregnancy but cannot conceive—and you want to terminate yours? Are you sure?

The next chapter explores assisted reproduction. How the arrival of lab-produced embryos and pregnancies achieved by medical intervention have changed our perception of human reproduction—further challenging the role of women in their reproductive tasks.

Notes

(1)   https://www.guttmacher.org/report/abortion-worldwide-2017-executive-summary. Accessed 25 Apr 2019.
(2)   Preventing unsafe abortion 26 June 2019. https://www.who.int/news-room/fact-sheets/detail/preventing-unsafe-abortion. Accessed 25 Aug 2019.
(3)   https://www.worldometers.info/abortions/.
(4)   Interactive map Center for reproductive rights. The World's Abortion Laws. https://reproductiverights.org/worldabortionlaws. Accessed 25 Aug 2019.
(5)   https://www.ansirh.org/research/global-turnaway-study. Accessed 2 Feb 2019.
(6)   https://bmcinthealthhumrights.biomedcentral.com/articles/10.1186/s12914-018-0174-2#Fn2. Accessed 12 Feb 2019.
(7)   https://www.guttmacher.org/fact-sheet/induced-abortion-worldwide. Accessed 12 Feb 2019.
(8)   https://www.guttmacher.org/report/abortion-worldwide-2017-executive-summary. Accessed 25.4.2019.
(9)   https://www.guttmacher.org/abortion-legality-worldwide. Accessed 25 Apr 2019.
(10)   https://www.guttmacher.org/state-policy/explore/overview-abortion-laws. Accessed 25 Apr 2019.
(11)   https://www.nytimes.com/interactive/2019/us/abortion-laws-states.html. Accessed 25 July 2019.
(12)   https://www.landmarkcases.org/cases/roe-v-wade. Accessed 25 Apr 2019.
(13)   https://legaldictionary.net/griswold-v-connecticut/. Accessed 11 Apr 2022.
(14)   Planned Parenthood v. Casey, 505 U.S. 833, 848–849 (1992). https://constitution.org/1-Constitution/2ll/2ndcourt/supreme/1sup.htm. Accessed 13 Apr 2022.
(15)   Planned Parenthood of Southeastern Pa. v. Casey, 505 U.S. 833 (1992). https://supreme.justia.com/cases/federal/us/505/833/. Accessed 13 Apr 2022.
(16)   Justice Scalia, joined by the Chief Justice White, and Justice Tomas. Planned Parenthood of Southeastern Pa. v. Casey, 505 U.S. 833 (1992). https://supreme.justia.com/cases/federal/us/505/833/ 841(7). Accessed 13 Apr 2022.
(17)   https://www.cbs.gov.il/he/mediarelease/pages/2019/פנינת-עוולת-הלספקת-היריה-ווייר-בשנים-2018-2017.aspx. Accessed 1 Aug 2019.
(18)   http://www.family-laws.co.il/divorce-jewish-couples-mens-tactics. Accessed 1 Aug 2019.
(19)   http://www.jewfaq.org/divorce.htm. Accessed 1 Aug 2019.
(20)   https://www.who.int/reproductivehealth/publications/preventing-unsafe-abortion-evidence-brief/en/. Accessed 1 Aug 2019.
(21)   https://www.opensocietyfoundations.org/explainers/what-global-gag-rule. Updated April 2019. Accessed 1 Feb 2020.
(22)   Center for Reproductive Rights. https://reproductiverights.org/. Accessed 18 Apr 2022.
(23)   https://bmcinthealthhumrights.biomedcentral.com/articles/10.1186/s12914-018-0183-1.
(24)   https://www.ansirh.org/sites/default/files/publications/files/turnaway_study_brief_web.pdf. Accessed 5 Feb 2020.
(25)   http://bit.ly/TurnawayStudy. Accessed 1 Feb 2020.

References

Eig, Jonathan. 2014. *The Birth of the Pill*. London: Macmillan.

Gay, Roxana. 2014. *Bad Feminist*. London: Corsair.

Jacobson, Thomas W., and W. Robert Johnston. 2018. *Abortion Worldwide Report, 1 Century, 100 Nations, 1 Billion Babies*. http://www.johnstonsarchive.net/policy/abortion/wrjp3318.html. Last modified 31 Dec 2018. Accessed 25 Apr 2019.

Johnson, B.R., A.F. Lavelanet, and S. Schlitt. 2018. Global abortion policies database: A new approach to strengthening knowledge on laws, policies, and human rights standards. *BMC International Health and Human Rights* 18: 35. https://doi.org/10.1186/s12914-018-0174-2.Accessed2.2.2019.

Kamin, Debra. 2014. Israel's Abortion Law Now Among World's Most Liberal. *The Times of Israel*. https://www.timesofisrael.com/israels-abortion-law-now-among-worlds-most-liberal/. Accessed 1 Aug 2019.

Lavelanet, A.F., S. Schlitt, B.R. Johnson, et al. 2018. Global Abortion Policies Database: A Descriptive Analysis of the Legal Categories of Lawful Abortion. *BMC International Health and Human Rights* 18: 44. https://doi.org/10.1186/s12914-018-0183-1.

Ramaswamy, C. 2019. Afterbirth. In *Nasty Women*, ed. Laura Jones, and Heather McDaid. London: 404 Ink.

Rogers, Adam. 2019. *Abortion Bans Create a Public Health Nightmare*. https://www.wired.com/story/abortion-bans-create-a-public-health-nightmare/. Accessed 25 July 2019.

Rose, Jacqueline. 2019. *Mothers. An Essay of Love and Cruelty*. London: Faber & Faber.

Sharon, Jeremy. 2019. *The Jerusalem Post*. www.jpost.com/Israel-News/As-abortion-fight-heats-up-in-US-termination-in-Israel-easily-accessible-589923. Accessed 1 Aug 2019.

World Health Organization (WHO). 2011. *Unsafe Abortion: Global and Regional Estimates of the Incidence of Unsafe Abortion and Associated Mortality in 2008*, 6th ed. Geneva: WHO. Accessed 25 Apr 2019.

Chapter 7
Assisted Reproduction Technologies (ARTs)

Whether to spare his patients anxiety, or to avoid scaring them off, or simply because he believed in the eventual success, Steptoe spun his version of the truth the way clinicians-investigators often did and still do: he accentuated the positive. (Robin Marantz-Henig 2004, p. 134)

More than four decades have passed since the birth of Louise Brown, the first child born as a result of in vitro fertilization (IVF) in 1978 (Steptoe and Edwards 1978) and, today, it is difficult to imagine the world without assisted reproductive technologies (ART). Indeed, despite much initial resistance by the medical community and by society, IVF has now firmly established its place in the clinical management of infertility (Revel 2009). In 2018 it was reported that 8 million IVF babies had been born in the 40 years since the historic first case in 1978,[1],[2],[3] ARTs have clearly affected both reproductive practices and our view of reproduction, in general. IVF has further medicalized and technologized reproduction, and although its development has increased procreative liberties, it has also reduced some people's freedom (Holm 2009). IVF has remained a challenging process for the women involved, and notwithstanding the low success rate, women, worldwide, subject themselves massively to the procedure.[1] This chapter provides a brief description of IVF from a medical perspective and examines some aspects of its history—the social, scientific, and political background in which it developed. Furthermore, this chapter focuses on the depiction and promotion of IVF in the present, and finally, asks whether women are coerced into IVF.

---

[1] I focus here on developed countries. For a discussion of IVF in developing countries see, Part II. Mind the Gap: Simonstein F. and Balanova K. Can't afford it, can't avoid it. Assisted reproduction in Israel and Bulgaria; Vayena, E. Assisted reproduction in developing countries: the debate at a turning point; Polack de Fried, E. Ethical and socio-cultural aspects that influence ART in Latin America. In, Frida Simostein (Ed) Reprogen-Ethics and the Future of Human Reproduction (2009). Springer.

95
F. Simonstein, *Womb Politics: A Short History of the Future of Human Reproduction*, The International Library of Bioethics 99, https://doi.org/10.1007/978-3-031-11654-4_6

7.1   IVF in a Nutshell

Fertilization may occur naturally after a heterosexual encounter when a sperm penetrates an egg inside the female body. IVF, by contrast, occurs in a Petri dish in the lab, where eggs retrieved from a woman's ovary and a man's sperm are placed together. The man collects sperm for IVF comfortably by himself whereas harvesting the eggs from the woman for IVF is challenging. It requires hormonal injections, first, followed by general anesthesia to retrieve the eggs from the ovaries. According to medical accounts, controlled ovarian stimulation (COS) induces the superovulation required to obtain several eggs for fertilization. Tailoring ovarian stimulation to the individual patient is challenging because ovarian response is considerably variable. This individual variability in ovarian response to COS requires dose adjustment "by strict patient monitoring." While exaggerated ovarian response might result in ovarian hyper stimulation syndrome (OHSS), if too few eggs are obtained, pregnancy rates may decrease. Moreover, the likelihood of pregnancy in a woman undergoing COS is subject to a large number of factors other than ovarian reserve and ovarian response (Revel 2009). The first three rounds with IVF (if the woman does not conceive) serve as an indication of how the woman responds to the IVF procedure (personal communication). In fact, each woman in the hands of an IVF expert becomes a new experimentation (see also Chap. 7).

If eggs are successfully retrieved for IVF and a sperm in the Petri dish penetrates the egg, fertilization occurs—outside the woman's body—and the first cell of an embryo is formed. After producing a few cells in the Petri dish, the embryo is returned to the woman's body and if it does implant in the womb, a new pregnancy begins. However, the zygote intrafallopian transfer (ZIFT)—the medical term for the technique of transferring embryos into the woman's fallopian tubes—is one area recognized as very challenging in IVF success rate because of the crucial role of endometrial receptivity. Indeed, ZIFT remains the trickiest stage in IVF since, although high quality embryos can be obtained in many patients, two out of three of such embryos will not implant in utero. Ariel Revel, an expert on IVF at the Hadassah IVF Unit in Jerusalem commented that "it is surprising that the human endometrium is so hostile to embryo implantation during most of the month. The exception lasts about two days and is termed the 'window of implantation.'" (Revel 2009). In fact, even after four decades since its first success, IVF has remained a challenging procedure (Zhou et al. 2008; Barash et al. 2003; Simon et al. 2003; Revel et al. 2005; Achache and Revel 2006).

7.2   Some Historical Aspects of IVF

In her book Pandora's Baby, Robin Marantz Henig remarks that today, when IVF is so routine that it is covered by health insurance in many countries, it is hard to believe that, in 1973, some viewed the procedure as a threat to "the very fabric of civilization." (Marantz-Henig 2004, p. 45).

Social Background

A Harris poll in 1969 found that more than half of American adults believed that the emerging reproductive technologies—in vitro fertilization, artificial insemination, and surrogate motherhood—were against God's will and would encourage promiscuity. More than two-thirds thought these techniques would signify "the end of babies born through love." Public sentiment was similar in Great Britain, where many people thought that fertilization of a human egg in the laboratory "was crossing a critical red line." (Marantz-Henig 2004, p. 50). These sentiments were described by Marantz-Henig:

> Marriage, fidelity, the essence of the family; our sense of who we are and where are we headed; what it means to be human, connected, normal, acceptable; ideas about love, sex, and nurturance; the willingness to yield to the inscrutable, marvellous mystery of it all. If in vitro fertilization was allowed, some said, all the stabilizing threads would unravel. (Marantz-Henig 2004, p. 6)

By the 1970s, other reproductive revolutions were taking place. The birth control pill had already separated sex from procreation (see Chap. 4); the Roe v. Wade decision had already separated pregnancy from childbirth (see Chap. 5), and no-fault divorce laws had already separated the "forever" component from marriage vows. All these coincident changes in the 1970s led to worries about what the new reproductive technology would do to people's perception of children "as the fruit of a loving, lifelong union"[4] (Justice Secretary Today 2019).

Women in the 1970s

Adding to these changes, women in the early 1970s were rewriting their social roles, moving out of housewifery, delaying childbearing or choosing to be childless altogether, and demanding access to traditionally male domains. In addition, the so-called leftists, at that time, said that it was a sorry thing to bring children into this world, the environmentalists said that more babies would further despoil the planet, and the feminists said that marriage as an institution "was sexist and suffocating." (Marantz-Henig 2004).

However, at the other end of the spectrum, millions of women remained "zealously pursuing" the traditional roles of mother and wife. While the emerging social movements of the early 1970s were undermining those very roles, millions of women still had no interest in reading books such as The Female Eunuch or The Second Sex, and wanted nothing more in their lives than to stay at home and raise their children. Marantz-Henig, for example, quotes Leslie Brown in an interview: "I longed for all those things that mothers usually moan about, like coping with dirty nappies and being kept awake all night." (Marantz-Henig 2004, p. 133). Indeed, women experiencing infertility was the background in which IVF could develop.

Political Background

In 1972, a British magazine ran a cover story suggesting that test tube babies were "the biggest threat since the atomic bomb" and demanding that the public rein in "the unpredictable scientists." (Marantz-Henig 2004, p. 86). In the United States, the government refused to sponsor IVF research. No government grants for in vitro fertilization meant that no one was forced to adhere to any standards. The research that Edwards and Steptoe were carrying out in England could not have been pursued in the United States—at least not with government money. It was not explicitly outlawed, but was not encouraged, either. Any American scientists who were studying in vitro fertilization were supporting their research with private money or with some clever rearrangement of grants for studies in a closely related field.

The problem with this approach was that IVF research would have benefited from the openness and coherence that federal funding would have provided. Scientists would have been forced to make their results known in a public forum, and grantees would have talked to each other and shared their experimental ups and downs. Federal funding also would have forced researchers to adhere to certain standards in order to receive their grants. However, IVF was a political risk, as highly organized antiabortionist forces and conservative groups had made the issue so charged that bureaucrats did what they could to steer clear of it (Marantz-Henig 2004).

Scientific Background

Entrepreneurial scientists were doing IVF boosted by private money from infertile couples who were "desperate" for babies of their own. Marantz Henig observes that many of these scientists were decent men and women with solid reputations and the loftiest of goals. Nevertheless, some were motivated by factors that drive many innovators and scientists: "ego, curiosity, ambition, even greed." These scientists were "free agents" who, in fact, did whatever they wanted and whatever the market would bear. As reported by Marantz Henig: "privately funded efforts turned some aspects of IVF into a cowboy science driven by supply and demand." (Marantz-Henig 2004, p. 12). Scientists pursuing IVF did have some inkling about the subject. However, this clearly constituted experimentation on human subjects without the subjects' knowledge. Leslie Brown, for example, realized that she was the first woman to become pregnant through IVF when reporters started to chase her. Steptoe and Edwards did not trouble to tell her that she was a first.

The Del Zio Case

In the United States, on July 18, 1978, the New York Times published an article titled "2 Charge ealous' [sic] Doctor Killed 'Test-Tube Baby,'" reporting that lawyers for a Florida couple who had sought to produce a "test-tube baby" five years previously charged in court that a physician at the Columbia Presbyterian Medical Center had deliberately destroyed a laboratory-fertilized embryo "because of poor relations between him and the physician who initiated the project."[5]

The story goes that Doris Del Zio could not have a baby because her fallopian tubes had been blocked. In September 1973, she underwent an operation at New York

Hospital to remove eggs from her ovarian tissue, and the eggs were then taken to the Columbia Presbyterian Medical Center and fertilized in a test tube with her husband's sperm by Dr. Landrum Shettles. He then stored the test tube in an incubator. The following day, Dr. Raymond Vande Wiele, Head of the Department, opened the test tube, thereby destroying the embryo.[6]

John and Doris Del Zio brought a civil suit against the medical center and against Vande Wiele, the physician who was chief of obstetrics and gynecology when the embryo was destroyed (Powledge 1978). The Del Zio couple asked for $1.5 million in damages on the ground that this action by Dr. Vande Wiele and the medical center had caused them "severe physical and mental anguish."[5] The prosecution charged that Vande Wiele had disliked Shettles and that this friction was behind his action. Vander Wiele's defense argued that Shettles had a poor record at the medical center, that he had been demoted often, and was not qualified for the experiment; that the methods used by the Del Zios' physicians were "scientifically unsound;" that they had no way of knowing whether their efforts would produce a "monster birth" or a normal child, and, that this was the physicians' "quest for glory" in which the Del Zio couple "were pawns" in a "genetic manipulation" procedure.[5]

Representatives of the medical center contended that the experiment was clandestine, that it violated the institution's regulations, and that it posed safety hazards for the woman in whose womb the embryo was to have been implanted. They said that the proposed endeavor posed the medical profession with larger questions of ethics and scientific standards—questions that were beyond the experimenters' coping capacity. However, the Del Zio case was in process when Lesley Brown, in England, was expected to give birth to "the first human fertilized within the artificial environment of a laboratory."[5]

Louise Brown was born on the seventh day of the Del Zio trial, and despite the judge's instruction to the jury to disregard this fact, it could not be ignored. The defense could no longer argue that IVF was impossible; a fool's dream. Consequently, the jury ruled against Vande Wiele, Columbia, and Columbia-Presbyterian, saying that they had engaged in behavior that was "utterly intolerable in a civilized community." The Del Zio couple won the case but were awarded only a fraction of the amount sought: $50,000 in damages to Doris and just $3 to John (Powledge 1978; The Del-Zios' Lawsuit 1978).

The First IVF Baby in the United States

Only in 1981, three years after the birth of Louise Brown, Elizabeth Carr was the first IVF baby born in the United States. Howard and Georgeanna Jones, both fertility experts at John Hopkins in Baltimore, who moved to Norfolk, Virginia, postponing retirement, had opened the first IVF clinic in the US. The Joneses had arrived in Norfolk on the day Louise Brown was born in England. In 1980, they had retrieved eggs from 41 women, had fertilized them successfully, transferred to the uterus 23 times, but had not achieved a single pregnancy.[7]

Since nothing they were doing was working, they decided to put the patients on strong fertility drugs to produce more eggs. Finally, while attending a conference in Paris, in the spring of 1981, the Joneses learned of the clinic's first pregnancy, but after celebrating, they prayed. In the end, Judy Carr gave birth to a girl, America's first test tube baby[8] (Frellick 2015). Nonetheless, just like Robert Edwards had prepared back in 1978, Howard Jones also had a written statement ready in his pocket about "the tragic news" and "the profound disappointment" (Marantz-Henig 2004, p. 225).

The Social Background Revisited

The most frightening thing about in vitro fertilization was the prospect of abnormal babies. Yet these fears rapidly fell away after Louise Brown, the first IVF baby, was born. She was normal. A poll taken in August 1978 after Louise Brown's birth, and directly after the verdict in the United States about "the first tube death trial" (the Del Zio trial), showed surprising acceptance of IVF. More than half of those polled said they would use IVF themselves if they were married and could not have a child. Two thirds of adults under 30 said they would try if they had to, and 60% of Americans thought IVF should be available for anyone who needed and wanted it.

Nonetheless, it was two years before the birth of the second baby with the aid of IVF—in 1980, in Australia, and three years before the third, in 1981, in the US. The fourth was born in France only in 1982.[9] The rest is history. However, just four successful births with IVF in four years is evidence of how challenging the IVF procedure was. It was the largest experiment on human subjects. The documented history of IVF does not include failed treatments throughout those years, nor how many women underwent the procedure unsuccessfully. We may suppose that there were many, many failed attempts and many, many disappointed women. Edwards and Steptoe, for example, had many failures with embryo transfer, rumoured to be anywhere from 60 to 200 unsuccessful tries.

7.3   IVF Today

In 2018, it was reported that 8 million IVF babies were born in the 40 years since the historic first case in 1978.[1],[3],[10],[9] Today, IVF may have become routine, but does not always guarantee success. In 2003, pregnancy from IVF was about 24% on average in the United States, according to the Centers for Disease Control and Prevention (CDC), and the birth rates were even lower (Marantz-Henig 2004). Worryingly, the success rate of IVF has not improved.

Present Success Rate

In 2017 and 2018, the success rate of IVF in the United States (according to the last CDC report) was 24.2 and 24%, respectively. Even more troubling is the fact that although the number of live births in 2018 compared with 2017 increased by 4923, and the rate of infants born with the aid of IVF in the US increased by 0.2%, the reason was that there were 21,812 more IVF cycles, an increase of 7.6% (Table 6.1).

This CDC report may not include success rates according to age (which decline with age; see Chap. 7) and with donor eggs (which improves the odds). However,

Table 6.1 CDC fertility clinic success rates report (https://www.cdc.gov/art/artdata/index.html. Accessed 2 Mar 2020)

	ART cycles	Reporting clinics	Live born infants	Success rate (%)	Live births (one or more infants)	More than one baby per delivery	Infants born with IVF (%)
2017	284,385	448	68,908	24.2	78,052	9144	1.7
2018	306,197	456	73,831	24.0	73,831	7647	1.9

since "successful" IVF clinics in the US are judged by their success rate, it is unlikely that mature women are admitted for the procedure. And the decision to pregnant using donor eggs is made after many failed attempts.[2]

The CDC rates above are not much different from Mother Nature's. They seem worse, however, because, as noted by Marantz-Henig, "the attempt itself affords no pleasure—only inconvenience, worry, discomfort, and expense." (Marantz-Henig 2004, p. 235). Despite the many uncertainties, she observes that IVF today seems to have a "Teflon reputation," as since the twenty-first century, IVF may be one of the first rather than the last steps on the fertility "merry-go-round." (Marantz-Henig 2004, p. 233). Today, IVF is considered a simple, necessary, and basically harmless procedure; a medical intervention with the same sorts of risks and benefits as any other intervention. In the words of Marantz Henig:

> Maybe the IVF patients' passion for babies makes them overlook the possible dangers of the path they have chosen. Or may they go to the enterprise with eyes wide open, having carefully considered their options and decided that IVF is worth the risk. (Marantz-Henig 2004, p. 242)

However, is any effort really made to open patients' (women's) eyes? Similarly to Steptoe and other scientists in the past, physicians today accentuate the positive. During the 1970s, it was generally left to scientists to choose what to tell—or not to tell—potential research subjects.

How Is IVF Presented in the 21st Century?

In 2006, a follow-up study in Israel was published, of 5310 cycles in a cohort of 1928 patients, claiming an 87% success rate following 14 consecutive cycles of IVF (Elizur et al. 2006). This gives an excellent impression, with only 13% of women supposedly failing to have a baby. We decided to analyze that study data further (Simonstein and Mashiach-Eizenberg 2012). Our analysis showed that only 35.7% of all the patients in the chosen cohort succeeded in having a baby, and that the rate of success per cycle was approximately 13%. The trend however, was—and remains—to blame failure on women for stopping treatment. As this is unlikely to happen in

---

[2] Interestingly, the idea and performance of donor eggs shows that women are not driven by genetics. They do not necessarily want a child who carries their genes. If so, what exactly stops women from adopting a child who already exists? The answer here would be that women desire to fulfill their female role: being pregnant. Yet another way for women to become mothers is through surrogacy. Thus, it seems that "anything goes" as long as IVF is involved.

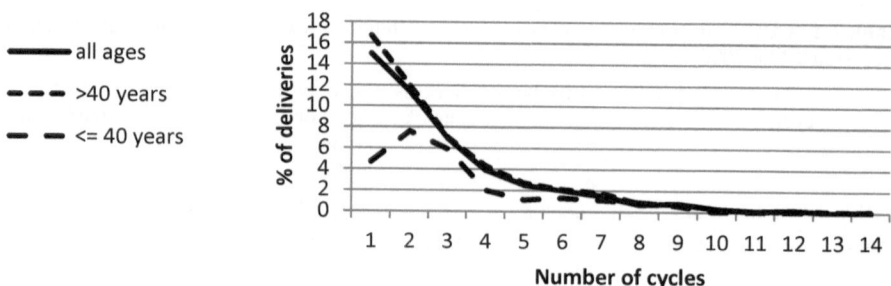

Fig. 6.1 % of new deliveries per IVF cycle calculated from "cumulative delivery rates" Simonstein and Mashiach-Eizenberg (2012)

the Israeli context because women are entitled to almost unlimited rounds with IVF for up to two children, even if they already have living children, that study assumed that after failed attempts in one clinic, women would move to another clinic and that non-returning women would succeed somewhere else.

Therefore, they recalculated an "estimated cumulative rate" to attain "a better measure of ultimate success." (Elizur et al. 2006). The graph was drawn optimistically in an upward direction. However, a closer examination of the figures in that study still revealed a familiar pattern: the three first cycles of IVF have the best chance, with success rates rapidly plummeting to zero after each new unsuccessful cycle. The cumulative rate between the third and the fourth cycle of IVF improved by just 4.4%, between the fourth and the fifth cycle by 2.7%, and so on; between the seventh and the eighth cycle, the odds for a live delivery dropped to 0.8%. Between the eighth and fourteenth cycles, the odds of having a baby with IVF are 0.1% (per cycle). Over the age of 40 it was zero (Fig. 6.1).

Thus, presenting a 90% "cumulative success rate" of IVF is misleading. Indeed, many women believe that if they stay in treatment, their chances of having a baby will *surely* improve (Remennick 2009). Yet in the aforementioned study (Elizur et al. 2006), while 604 women succeeded in having a baby, 1234 did *not*. The authors of that study then asked: "How far should we go?" They promptly answered this question by telling the story of two couples who conceived after 18 and 23 cycles. They continued: "... although these situations are rare, it is still possible to succeed, even after such a high order of treatments." (Elizur et al. 2006). In other words, they were suggesting that women continue endlessly with IVF for the sake of a miraculous event. Troublingly, these rare events are accentuated by the media, adding to the misleading idea that perseverance with IVF is the ultimate option to succeed in having a baby.

What Clinics Tell Prospective Patients (i.e., Women)

Imprecise advertisement of IVF is due not only to the positive but misleading outlook of its success described in professional papers. When addressing prospective clients (women), IVF clinics present the procedure as being as close as possible to the natural process. Indeed, the word "natural" appears several times, suggesting that the process is not as artificial as it may seem. The website of the Monash IVF clinic,[11] which is one example among many, starts off by explaining that one round of IVF treatment begins on the first day of the menstrual period, with the onset of hormone injections to stimulate the ovaries. It continues to explain that in a "natural monthly cycle," a woman's ovaries normally produce one egg, but the woman in IVF treatment will be injected with medication, either once or twice throughout the 28-day cycle, or one to two per day for eight to 14 days, to encourage the follicles in her ovaries to produce more eggs "that are already there."

The website explains further that the most common hormones in the medications (FSH and LH) "are produced *naturally* in the body," to boost "the *natural* levels to encourage more eggs to develop." A trigger injection would render the eggs ready for ovulation, which is "the *natural process*" where eggs are released and the woman has her period. Egg retrieval will be scheduled prior to ovulation. The website remarks also that egg retrieval in which the eggs are collected from the woman's ovaries "takes just around 20–30 min" and that after recovery, "the woman will be able to walk out on her own." It adds almost as an afterthought that "she would need to have a support person with her as she won't be able to drive after the procedure." The fact that egg retrieval takes place under general anesthesia is an under-emphasized detail on the website.

What happens next? According to the explanation, following the retrieval proce-dure, the eggs and some sperm are placed in a dish. If the sperm fertilizes the egg, it becomes an embryo. Then the embryo is placed in a special incubator "where the conditions for growth and development are perfect." Not all eggs will fertilize and reach embryo stage, however. "The eggs might not be mature or the sperm not be strong enough." If the embryo does develop in the lab, the woman is then ready for it to be transferred into her uterus.According to the fertility clinic website, the embryo transfer "is a very simple process, like a pap smear;" stressing that "it takes about 5 min," "the woman will be awake"…"there's no anesthetic," and "she can get up straight away."

This sounds very nice and easy. However, this is the ZIFT procedure which, as noted above, is the trickiest part of IVF, as it does not work in the majority of cases (approximately 85% failure rate). This detail does not appear on the fertility clinic website. On the contrary, the explanation continues smoothly: "about two weeks after the embryo transfer, she will have a blood test to measure the levels of the human chorionic gonadotropin (hCG) hormone. hCG in her bloodstream usually means a positive pregnancy test."[11] To sum up, the clinic website makes the IVF process look very easy, simple, and natural—but is this true?

First, the whole process is not as natural as the attempted portrayal on the website. Nowhere does it say that the "natural" substances are injected *in excess* to mature more eggs than normal, to produce *over-ovulation*. In the IVF retrieval procedure, the average number of eggs is between eight and 15. In the natural process, usually, only one egg matures. Second, egg retrieval is a stage in IVF that must be performed under general anesthesia. This is not stressed on the website and usually not acknowledged very much by the general public. Furthermore, the insertion of embryos back into the woman—ZIFT—does not work in approximately 85% of IVF cycles. Finally, the overall success rate of IVF remains at around 25–40%. Thus, more than half the women in IVF treatment would remain childless, and worse off than when they started with IVF (Remennick 2009).

7.4   ART at All Cost for Women?

Even without IVF, a pregnancy is risky. Pregnancy symptoms and complications can range from mild and annoying discomfort to severe, sometimes life-threatening, illnesses.[12],[13] Two out of every five pregnancies have difficulties along the way. The risks of a pregnancy include inter alia high blood pressure, gestational diabetes, severe, persistent nausea and vomiting, anemia, preeclampsia. Preeclampsia is a serious condition that can lead to preterm delivery and death.[13] Preeclampsia can cause high blood pressure and damage to one or more organs, often the kidneys (causing protein in the urine). It occurs in about 7% of all pregnancies.In Australia, for example, preeclampsia affects about 15,000 pregnant women every year.[14],[15],[16],[17]

So, if women are willing to put themselves at risk with natural pregnancies, why should they worry about IVF? The answer to this question is that IVF carries higher risk and yet, to achieve a pregnancy, it seems that anything goes. Pergonal, for example, was a powerful fertility drug used in 1981, which caused mood swings and irritability and occasionally led to masculinizing side effects including increased hair growth and deepening of the voice (Revel 2009). Pergonal has since been replaced by other fertility hormones that still have mild to life-threatening side effects. In addition, the long-term hazards of these fertility drugs have remained controversial. A review from the *Cochrane Database,* in 2017, concluded that the synthesis of the available evidence did not allow the drawing of robust conclusions, "due to the very low quality of evidence." Moreover, the review concluded that the "evidence regarding exposure to gonadotropins [fertility hormones] was inconclusive." (Skalkidou et al. 2017). The *Cochrane Database* conclusions are hardly surprising, since most of the IVF research is funded and promoted by the IVF industry.

In addition to higher health risks with the pregnancy, women undergoing treatment with IVF face a 20-fold increased risk of twins and a 400-fold increased risk of higher order pregnancies (triplets or more) (Martin and Welch 1998). Multiple pregnancies, including twins, is not a desirable outcome of IVF treatment as it carries an increased risk of very serious consequences, including premature birth and cerebral palsy. Having only a single embryo transferred could prevent these complications (Revel 2009). This may not occur if clinics are ethical and limit transfer.

Conveniently, the European Society of Human Reproduction (ESHRE) and Embryology and the American Society for Reproductive Medicine (ASRM) have included ethics discussions in their format. For example, at the forthcoming ESHRE congress in 2022, there is a session for and against emerging technologies. Following this session will be a one-hour SIG Ethics and Law members' meeting (special interest group). Of course, it is ideal that this SIG exists within the ESHRE; and the ethics discussions are welcomed. The trouble is that the ethics debates at the ESHRE remain at the debatable point until the new technology takes over. At the end of the day, the main interest and preoccupation of ESHRE and ASRM is with "reproduction."[3] And the ethics deliberations do not exactly focus on women beyond their "need" to reproduce.[4]

And so, despite awareness of the risks of twins, patients, as well as practitioners, have remained uncertain about adopting a single embryo transfer policy in routine clinical practice and continue to question its clinical and cost effectiveness (Pandian et al. 2005). At the end of the day, clinics are subject to success rates and transferring more than one has higher probability of success. Another reason to transfer more than one is that "women want so much to be pregnant…" (Personal communication).

Another challenge imposed by IVF was placing further strain on the marital relationship by depersonalizing one of its most intimate acts, in addition to the time, expense, and the odds against it even working. So why do women still (massively) submit themselves to IVF? According to Marantz-Henig, despite all the negatives of IVF, a couple might reasonably conclude that the risks are worth it for the sake of the big payoff—having a baby of their own:

> A baby will bring great joy to the marriage, the odds of having a normal baby through IVF outweighs the odds of having a damaged one, many of the problems uncovered in some studies, such as low birth weight, could be mild and adoption is a difficult process. (Marantz-Henig 2004, p. 243)

However, whereas IVF may mean salvation for some women, it may mean imprisonment for others.

Are Women Coerced into ART?

According to Holm (2009), the increase in procreative liberties created by the developments of ARTs has indirectly decreased the freedom of some people (i.e., women). This situation has come about because the broad social acceptance of IVF in many countries has changed social default expectations with regard to reproductive choices. Holm observes that anyone who admits to being infertile and still has some desire for children "is likely to be met with the expectation that they should engage in

---

[3] For example, the ESHRM international congress to be held in 2022 in Milan reads as follows: "We are hopeful that you can all join us for our Annual Meeting to celebrate the world's largest in-person event in *reproductive science and medicine*. And once again, for this 2022 edition, ESHRE will offer an irresistible *scientific programme*, which includes a wide range of precongress courses, inspiring presentations on current key topics, selected presentations of *new research, industry sponsored symposia* and lively networking opportunities" (my italics). https://www.eshre.eu/ESHRE2022/Home/Welcome-to-Milan. Accessed 10 Apr 2022.

[4] The "Controversies in reproductive genetics" (Part 1) session will discuss pre-implantation genetic tests (PGT) for "polygenic risks scores," "mitochondrial replacement therapies," "genome editing in the human embryo" and "Uterine Lavage for PGT on in vivo produced embryos." The "ethics" talks would be replies to presentations defending an emerging technology. There is room to hope that the last item—that includes the word "uterine" in its title—might refer to "women" in its "ethical considerations." The other items do not. https://www.eshre.eu/ESHRE2022/Home/Welcome-to-Milan. Accessed 10 Apr 2022.

ART treatment." According to Holm, this will lead some people, "a minority," to pursue such treatments "against their own better judgment," and "may negatively affect the wellbeing of a much larger group who will feel under pressure to defend their decision not to use ART." (Holm 2009).

Nonetheless, the argument that women are socially coerced into using ART and that this is a good reason to ban ART is controversial. Alan Petersen, for example, rejects this argument, mainly because there is no good reason to believe that the choices in question are not autonomous. As part of his rejection, Petersen states that if women are being coerced to desire to use ART, we should eradicate the coercive elements in pronatalist ideology, not access to ART (Petersen 2004). Against this conclusion, Soren Holm argues that this is a version of a common argument in bioethics, stating that if a certain negative effect of an act or policy can be traced to some kind of prejudice or ideology in society, that is not a reason not to perform the act or not to introduce the policy, but is a reason to eradicate the prejudice or ideology. According to Holm, however, it is seldom explicated how such an eradication should be achieved, or who might be responsible for achieving it. Holm suggests breaking free from this norm in bioethics and questions "how the negative effects of ART on some people's freedom and welfare can be ameliorated or eradicated, and who might be responsible in this context." (Holm 2009).

Who, indeed, is responsible? This question has remained unanswered.

In the meantime, a thriving ARTs industry has developed, and pressurizing women over reproduction, as a woman's duty, continues.[5] Some politicians and the Pope have been quoted as saying that women who do not have children "are selfish."[6] Some scientific reports also blame women for the low success rate with IVF. They claim that the low success rate with IVF reflects the trend toward delaying the birth of a first child until an age at which female fecundity or reproductive capacity has been lowered and this has increased the incidence of age-related infertility. This happens because in about half of the IVF cycles reported in Europe and America, the woman is 35 years of age or older, reflecting this demographic trend. According to these reports, "IVF by itself cannot compensate for the lower fecundity associated with increasing age;" so expectations from IVF should, therefore, be realistic: "Women should realize that although IVF is a very strong tool, its efficacy drops after age 35 and plummets after age 40." (Andersen et al. 2008; Wright et al. 2004; Baird et al. 2005).

Following these reports about women pursuing IVF later in life, Daniel Callahan, then at the Hastings Center, and Renzo Pegoraro, academic adviser to the Pope,[(18)] both renowned bioethicists, proposed—separately—that women should have children first, and only then go to college (or university) to pursue a career (personal communication). Callahan cites his wife as an example (Callahan and Simonstein 2009). I, myself, am an example of the same thing. Like Callahan's wife, I did my university degrees, including my PhD, only after I had had two children. However,

---

[5] For instance, lesbian women in Israel are more accepted by society after having a child.

[6] This is not to say that the Pope favors IVF. He does not.

clearly, we are the exceptions. For even women who already have a career have difficulty climbing the ladder to higher positions. Most women would not go to college or university after having children, as child care remains mostly the mother's job (see Chap. 1).

7.5 Conclusions

More than four decades have passed since the first child was born as a result of IVF in 1978. Despite much initial resistance by the medical community and by society, IVF has become the first rather than the last option for treating infertility. IVF was developed during a time when women were attaining freedom from unwanted pregnancies, with the development of the pill, and the legalization of abortion. Nonetheless, stories of infertile women "desperately" wanting children and pursuing IVF brought back the idealization of a maternal vocation that every "normal" woman must have. Infertile women wanting children and doing IVF became publicly applauded.

The development of IVF was the largest experiment on human subjects and seems to have remained experimental. Although treatment of infertility with IVF has increased enormously, the overall rate of success with IVF cycles has remained painfully low (see also Chap. 7). Less than 50% of women will achieve a pregnancy with IVF, and even fewer will get a take-home baby. In addition, IVF is riskier than a natural pregnancy, and the long-term dangers remain unclear. IVF is advertised in an utterly optimistic and misleading manner, but has nevertheless developed a Teflon reputation, and is promoted by a thriving industry.

In the context of womb politics, IVF has further medicalized and technologized reproduction, and whereas this development in developed countries has increased procreative liberties for some, IVF has also reduced the freedom of others (while in developing countries, IVF remains inaccessible). In developed societies, women might feel free to (not) commit themselves to IVF, if they do (not) want to. However, even in these countries, women may still feel obligated to use the procedure, since it exists. The pressure on women to reproduce, marketed as "this is what women do and want," persists. It has been suggested that the societal factors coercing women to reproduce should be addressed, and not IVF. However, the question of whether women are coerced into IVF has remained largely unanswered. Moreover, under the present demographic negative growth in developed countries, childless women are considered "selfish."

Furthermore, in pronatalist societies, women do not seem to have much escape from IVF, even more so if it is funded by the state. The next chapter presents the use—and misuse—of IVF in a developed country with a pronatalist society.

Notes

(1) https://www.nbcnews.com/health/health-news/million-babies-have-been-born-u-s-fertility. Accessed 1 Aug 2020.
(2) https://www.simplemost.com/at-least-8-million-ivf-babies-have-been-born-in-the-last-40-years. Accessed 1 Aug 2020.
(3) https://edition.cnn.com/2018/07/03/health/worldwide-ivf-babies-born-study/index.html. Accessed 1 Aug 2020.
(4) P:\Pub\Final Acts\Final Acts_YR\PRE80\UMDA 1973.wpd § 302a(2), p. 37. Accessed 8 July 2020.
(5) 2 Charge zealous' Doctor Killed 'Test-Tube Baby' July 18, 1978. Accessed 20 Aug 2020.
(6) https://www.nytimes.com/1978/07/18/archives/2-charge-jealous-doctor-killed-testtube-baby-15-million-damages.html. Accessed 20 Aug 2020.
(7) https://www.hopkinsmedicine.org/news/media/releases/howard_w_jones_jr_pioneer_in_reproductive_medicine_dies_at_104.
(8) Howard and Georgeanna Jones. https://www.pbs.org/wgbh/americanexperience/features/babies-bio-joness/. Accessed 2 Mar 2020.
(9) https://ivf-worldwide.com/ivf-history.html. Accessed 2.3.2020.
(10) Howard and Georgeanna Jones. https://www.pbs.org/wgbh/americanexperience/features/babies-bio-joness/. Accessed 2.3.2020.
(11) https://monashivf.com/fertility-treatments/fertility-treatments/the-ivf-process/. Accessed 20 Aug 2020.
(12) https://www.cdc.gov/reproductivehealth/maternalinfanthealth/pregnancy-complications.html. Accessed 1 Aug 2020.
(13) https://www.womenshealth.gov/pregnancy/youre-pregnant-now-what/pregnancy-complications. Accessed 1 Aug 2020.
(14) https://www.nichd.nih.gov/health/topics/pregnancy/conditioninfo/complications. Accessed 20 Aug 2020.
(15) https://www.mydr.com.au/babies-pregnancy/toxaemia-of-pregnancy. Accessed 1 Aug 2020.
(16) https://www.thelancet.com/journals/lancet/article/PIIS0140-6736(00)05215-6/fulltext. Accessed 1 Aug 2020.
(17) https://www.sciencedirect.com/topics/pharmacology-toxicology-and-pharmaceutical-science/toxemia. Accessed 1 Aug 2020.
(18) http://www.academyforlife.va/content/pav/en/the-academy/the-chancellor.html. Accessed 1 July 2020.

References

Achache, H., and A. Revel. 2006. Endometrial Receptivity Markers, The Journey to Successful Embryo Implantation. *Human Reproduction Update* 12 (6): 731–746.
Andersen, A.N., V. Goossens, A.P. Ferraretti, S. Bhattacharya, R. Felberbaum, J. de Mouzon, et al. 2008. Assisted Reproductive Technology in Europe, 2004: Results Generated from European Registers by ESHRE. *Human Reproduction* 23 (4): 756–771.
Baird, D.T., J. Collins, J. Egozcue, L.H. Evers, L. Gianaroli, H. Leridon, et al. 2005. Fertility and Ageing. *Human Reproduction Update* 11 (3): 261–276.
Barash, A., N. Dekel, S. Fieldust, I. Segal, E. Schechtman, and I. Granot. 2003. Local Injury to the Endometrium Doubles the Incidence of Successful Pregnancies in Patients Undergoing in Vitro Fertilization. *Fertility and Sterility* 79 (6): 1317–22.
Callahan, D. 2009. Women, Work, and Children: Is There a Solution? In *Reprogen-Ethics and the Future of Gender*, ed. Frida Simonstein, 91–104. London: Springer.

Elizur, S.E., L. Lerner-Geva, J. Levron, A. Shulman, D. Bider, and J. Dor. 2006. Cumulative Live Birth Rate Following in vitro Fertilization: Study of 5310 Cycles. *Gynecological Endocrinology* 22: 25–30.

Frellick, M. 2015. *Dr Howard Jones, Who Brought IVF to US, Dies at 104*. https://www.medscape.com/viewarticle/849249. Accessed 2 Dec 2015.

Henig, M.R. 2004. *Pandora's Baby*. NY: Houghton Mifflin.

Holm, Soren. 2009. The Medicalisation of Reproduction—A 30 Years Perspective. In *Reprogen-Ethics and the Future of Gender*, 29–36, ed. Frida Simonstein. London: Springer.

Justice Secretary Today. 2019. *Divorcing Couples Will No Longer have to Blame Each Other for the Breakdown of Their Marriage as the Justice Secretary Today (9 April 2019) Announced a New Law to Help Reduce Family Conflict*. https://www.gov.uk/government/news/new-divorce-law-to-end-the-blame-game. Accessed 1 July 2020.

Martin, P.M., and H.G. Welch. 1998. Probabilities for Singleton and Multiple Pregnancies After in vitro Fertilization. *Fertility and Sterility* 70 (3): 478–481.

Pandian, Z., A. Templeton, G. Serour, and S. Bhattacharya. 2005. Number of Embryos for Transfer After IVF and ICSI: A Cochrane Review. *Human Reproduction* 20 (10): 2681–2687.

Petersen, T.S. 2004. A Woman's Choice?—On Women, Assisted Reproduction and Coercion. *Ethical Theory and Moral Practice* 7: 81–90.

Powledge, T. 1978. A Report from the Del Zio Trial. *The Hastings Center Report* 8 (5): 15–17. https://doi.org/10.2307/3561442.

Remennick, L. 2009. Childless in the Land of Imperative Motherhood: Stigma and Coping Among Infertile Israeli Women. *Sex Roles* 43: 821–841.

Revel, Ariel. 2009. Current Status of Assisted Reproductive Techniques (ART)—A 30 Years Retrospective. In *Reprogen-Ethics and the Future of Gender*, ed. Frida Simonstein, 15–28. London: Springer.

Revel, A., A. Helman, M. Koler, A. Shushan, O. Goldshmidt, E. Zcharia, et al. 2005. Heparanase Improves Mouse Embryo Implantation. *Fertility and Sterility* 83 (3): 580–6.

Simonstein, F., and M. Mashiach-Eizenberg. 2012. How Long Should Women Persevere with IVF? *Journal of Health Services Research & Policy* 17 (2): 121–123.

Simon, A., A. Safran, A. Revel, E. Aizenman, B. Reubinoff, A. Porat-Katz, et al. 2003. Hyaluronic Acid Can Successfully Replace Albumin as the Sole Macromolecule in a Human Embryo Transfer Medium. *Fertility and Sterility* 79 (6): 1434–1438.

Skalkidou, A., T.N. Sergentanis, S.P. Gialamas, et al. 2017. Risk of Endometrial Cancer in Women Treated with Ovary-Stimulating Drugs for Subfertility. *The Cochrane Database of Systematic Reviews* 3 (3): CD010931. Published 25 Mar 2017. https://doi.org/10.1002/14651858.CD010931.pub2

Steptoe, P.C., and R.G. Edwards. 1978. Birth After the Reimplantation of a Human Embryo. *Lancet* 2 (8085): 366.

The Del-Zios' Lawsuit. 1978. *American Experience*. http://www.shoppbs.pbs.org/wgbh/amex/babies/peopleevents/e_suit.html. Accessed 20 Aug 2020.

Wright, V.C., J. Chang, G. Jeng, M. Chen, and M. Macaluso. 2007. Assisted Reproductive Technology Surveillance—United States, 2004. *MMWR Surveillance Summaries* 56 (6): 1–22.

Zhou, L., R. Li, R. Wang, H.X. Huang, and K. Zhong. 2008. Local injury to the endometrium in controlled ovarian hyperstimulation cycles improves implantation rates. *Fertility and Sterility* 89 (5): 1166–1176.

Chapter 8
Is IVF an Ongoing Experiment?

Reproductive hazards have traditionally been viewed as women's fate and as taken for granted. For instance, Cook, Dickens, and Fathalla explain that maternity is not a disease but "an essential function that women fulfill for the survival of our species." (Cook et al. 2003, p. 29). They remark, however, that although maternity is not a disease, pregnancy may compromise women's health and can sometimes be deadly. Indeed, the WHO reports that 300,000 women died from reproductive hazards in 2015.[1] Medical intervention in reproductive matters has saved many lives and has generally contributed to women's welfare.[1] The goal of saving the life of a pregnant woman and her baby has been extended to incorporate more sophisticated aims, such as helping a woman conceive in the first place, thus "curing" individuals and couples from numerous impediments to reproduction.

Celebrating 40 years of in vitro fertilization (IVF) in a special issue of the Fertility and Sterility journal, the editors equate the birth of the first IVF baby, in 1978, with the technological advance of humans walking on the moon (Niederberger and Pellicer 2018). Infertility, although a distressful condition, is not a disease and is certainly not a lethal threat to the individual. However, the medical profession has built it up as a "terrible disease." Forty years ago, a woman who could not have a child due to infertility could be "excused" from motherhood. She was probably unhappy for a while, but she could adopt a child or, alternatively, had the chance to get on with her life and perhaps engage in other things.

Today, in the era of ARTs, optional childlessness (mainly but not exclusively) in paternalistic societies has become (almost) unthinkable. For example, in 2004, the philosopher Matty Häyry suggested that couples should be advised that it is OK to remain childless (Hñyry 2004), but his proposal was not popular among his colleagues (Aksoy 2004; Bennet 2004; Holm 2004).

---

[1] Certainly since 1847, when Ignaz Semmelweis claimed that the incidence of puerperal fever could be drastically reduced by enforcing hand-washing among medical students and staff.

F. Simonstein, *Womb Politics: A Short History of the Future of Human Reproduction*,
The International Library of Bioethics 99,
https://doi.org/10.1007/978-3-031-11654-4_7

Marantz-Henig notes that many consider having children as a God-given right; others think of it as a right that is protected in the constitution. But the question of what takes precedence remains: society's right to keep its healthcare expenditures under control, or the couple's right to beget a child, through any possible means (Marantz-Henig 2004). Holm also observed that no healthcare system funds unlimited access to all ARTs legally available within that particular jurisdiction, and very few fund any access to ARTs that are legally available only outside the jurisdiction (Holm 2009). Holm seems unaware of what happens with ART in Israel, however.

Israel supports unlimited rounds of IVF up to two children; even if the woman has children already. This policy claims to support a "woman's need" to have babies; and, worldwide, Israel is regarded as the "North Star" for IVF policy. However, is this permissive IVF policy successful? To answer this question, empirical research is necessary. This chapter presents a version of a study on the effectiveness of the Israeli policy on IVF in two Israeli IVF clinics (Simonstein et al. 2014). It focuses on the open-ended Israeli policy on IVF, admired by many, and examines the social and political aspects behind this policy. Finally, this chapter asks whether IVF is an ongoing experiment.

8.1 IVF in Israel

In 2006, a paper published in the Fertility and Sterility journal noted that Israel provides 100% of "IVF optimal utilization." (Nachtigall 2006). That paper did not explicitly explain how "optimal" was calculated. We may suppose, however, that the definition derives from the highest number of IVF cycles supplied by any healthcare system, because Israel's National Health Insurance (NHI) covers unlimited cycles of IVF for *all* Israeli women for up to two children in a given relationship, even if the woman already has living children. A synonym of "optimal" is "best"—but are unlimited cycles of IVF really best? And if so, best for whom?

Rate of IVF Cycles and Effectiveness

Since the 1990s, the rate of IVF cycles in Israel has increased almost threefold among women in their fertile years.[2] According to the Israeli NHI, the increase in IVF cycles has been higher than the rate of population growth. In 2006, there were 15 cycles per 1000 women between the ages of 15 and 49 compared to 12 in 2000, and eight in 1995. In 2009, 4.2% of all live births in Israel were due to IVF, compared with 1.7% in 1995.[3] In 2017, the percentage of IVF births was 4.6, an increase of almost 10% since 2010. However, the number of IVF cycles in 2017 compared with the number of IVF cycles in 2010 increased by almost 37% (Table 8.1).

In 2012, we observed that the higher rate of live births was due to the increased number of cycles per woman and not to improved IVF treatment (Simonstein and Mashiach-Eizenberg 2012). This trend has persisted in Israel and in the United States (see Chap. 7). In Israel, the average success rate of IVF (rated by live births) has remained constant for the last two decades at 16–17% of live births per IVF cycle.

Table 8.1 Number of IVF cycles in Israel[3]

Year	Number of IVF cycles	Number of cycles per 1000 women	Percentage of IVF births
1995	5000	8	1.7
2000	18,000	12	2.6
2006	26,000	15	3.5
2010	31,978	17.8	4.2
2017	43,695	21.5	4.6[2]

Table 8.2 Percentage of success rate of IVF in Israel (rated by live births per cycle) 2000–2017[2]

2000	2002	2006	2007	2008	2009	2010	2011	2012	2013	2014	2015	2016	2017
15.5	17.9	16.8	17.2	16.0	16.7	16.2	14.9	16.3	15.7	16.5	18.0	17.8	17.1

Indeed, the success rate in 2017 was 17.1%, similar to the rate of success in 2006 and 2007 (16.8% and 17.2% respectively) and lower than the success rate in 2002 (17.9%). Furthermore, the rate of success in 2013 was similar to the rate of success in 2000 (15.7% and 15.5% respectively)[2] (Table 8.2).

How Many Rounds of IVF Do Women in Israel Undergo?

The statistics about IVF at the NHI present the number of IVF cycles per 1000 women aged 15–49. Inclusion of all women throughout their fertile years may be a global norm, but is misleading. According to the last population census by the Israeli CBS, in 2017, there were 333,800 girls aged 15–19 and 306,500 women aged 19–24.[4] Thus, more than half a million women who were far from procuring IVF were, nevertheless, still counted. No one in the 15–19 age group needs IVF, and it is pursued only rarely by the 19–24 age group. Hence the impossibility of knowing— from these data alongside an unlimited policy—how many IVF cycles are really performed per 1000 women in Israel.

The excuse given for this gap on this significant data is that Israeli women who do not succeed in one IVF unit go to another. It is argued that women starting in a new clinic are often untruthful about their previous IVF treatments (personal communication). So, according to such a concept, it is impossible to know how many rounds of IVF women in Israel really undergo. This is strange, because every Israeli citizen is issued with an identification number either at birth or on immigration to the country.[2] This individual identification number is used, for example, on driving licenses, bank accounts, and in crime detection. In health services also, every Israeli man, woman, and child must register this identification number prior to any healthcare procedure or when purchasing prescribed medication. This information is shared

---

[2] I am aware that in other countries, some people may be opposed to a nationwide civil identification number (personal communication). Yet in Israel, a personal number to identify people already exists, and it is not my intention here to discuss whether the system is good or bad.

among different pharmacies, providing a record of the prescribed drugs purchased and preventing repeated purchases without acquiring a new prescription.

This begs the question of why the number of IVF cycles that a woman does in one clinic cannot be traced in a similar manner in all the other IVF units in Israel, of which there are presently 26.[5] The data saved in one IVF unit are not shared with the other 25, supposedly because of patient privacy. Pharmacies, however, keep a record of drugs purchased in order to protect their customers, which certainly constitutes paternalistic care. Besides acknowledging the paternalistic nature of this tracing procedure, I cannot see any harm in it, though. If it is acceptable, then keeping track of the number of IVF rounds that a woman has undergone in Israel—to prevent her from concealing this information—would be a similar method of protecting her from damaging herself. Indeed, in a country that allows unlimited rounds of IVF, the number of IVF cycles a woman does is crucial for everyone.

How Many Babies Are Actually Born in Israel After Unsuccessful Cycles?

In the context of availability and access to IVF, many look upon the Israeli policy as the North Star (Damianov 2002; Simonstein and Balabanova 2009). But is the Israeli policy of endless rounds of IVF effective? As mentioned above, the number of IVF cycles a woman may undergo in Israel remains unknown because of the inauthentic data provided. The information on the Ministry of Health website shows the overall rate of success per cycle of IVF, but does not mention the cumulative rate of success by the number of cycles per woman. Hence the remaining question as to how many babies are actually born in Israel after many unsuccessful cycles.

The cumulative live birth rates with IVF, worldwide, are presented as very high (Malizia et al. 2009; Pelinck et al. 2008). Yet, overall, the rate of success after seven *failed* attempts is zero or almost zero (see also Chap. 7). This result raises the question of how many babies are actually born in Israel, with its limitless policy, after many unsuccessful cycles. To investigate this question, in 2010, my colleagues and I performed a retrospective analysis of whether the results and effectiveness of open-ended IVF justify the policy of limitless rounds (Simonstein et al. 2014). The following section presents a version of this research.

8.2   ART Policies in Israel: A Retrospective Analysis of IVF-Embryo Transfer

Materials and Methods

Research Sample

The research included 573 files reviewed during 2011–2013 in two IVF clinics, in central and northern Israel. These clinics were chosen because of the multicultural background of the surrounding population. The research sample consisted of the total number of women who started treatment in 2000 or were in treatment during 2010 in these two clinics (five clinics were approached initially; inclusion in this study was voluntary). From the 573 files reviewed, 38 were excluded due to incomplete information. In total, 535 files were included in the analysis.

The research sample was divided into two groups:

1. Women who started treatment with IVF in 2000 (thereafter the 2000 cohort) in these clinics (n = 210).
2. Women who were in treatment with IVF during 2010 in these clinics (n = 350). The year 2010 was chosen to examine some newer data.

The reason for choosing a cohort of patients from 2000 as the starting point of this study (2011) was twofold:

a. To track records from medical files during a decade, retrospectively, and
b. To ensure that the 2000 sample did not include women who could still be in treatment, as Remennick (2000) observed that women may persevere with IVF treatment for seven years or more.

The study included only non-donor cycles. Subgroups included age at start of treatment.

Data included demographic variables (year of birth, country of origin, personal status, number of children); physiological variables (blood count, blood pressure, weight, BMI), and variables about the treatment with IVF (number of cycles, duration of infertility, pregnancies, births, take home baby, number of hospitalizations during treatment). In both groups, most of the women were married (92%); most of the women were Jewish (78%); other women were Arab citizens including Muslims, Christians, and Druze.

IVF-Embryo Transfer Treatment

Gonadotropin releasing hormone (GnRH) analogue protocol, agonist or antagonist, and controlled ovarian hyper-stimulation were chosen on a case-to-case basis according to standard clinical practice. Conventional IVF and/or intra-cytoplasmic sperm injection (ICSI) were performed according to the cause of infertility (either the woman *or* the man had the problem). The number of embryos transferred was in accordance with national guidelines. Cryopreservation of supernumerary embryos was generally performed 48–72 days after oocyte (egg) retrieval. In frozen–thawed embryo transfer cycles, endometrial preparation was performed in accordance with the simplified approach with no GnRH analogue supplementation. The treatment was sequential, starting with estrogen to prime the endometrium till it reaches at least 8 mm thickness, measured by vaginal ultrasound, followed by estrogen and progesterone treatment for luteal support (Younis et al. 2008, 2013).

Statistical Analysis

Analyses were computed using the Predictive Analytics SoftWare (PASW, Version 18.0). Descriptive data on the study cohort, such as age at the start of treatment, number of treatments and cycles, and rates of success with IVF, were presented as absolute figures, rates, or percentages. Group comparisons were performed using *t*-test. Correlation between the number of treatments and the number of hospitalizations were performed using Pearson correlation. Significance was set at the 0.05 level, and all tests of significance were two-tailed.

Results

2000 Cohort

The average age at the start of the IVF treatment was 32.5 ($SD = 6.2$).

Number of Cycles and Treatments

Cycles: In this study, a cycle was noted at the egg/s retrieval stage. We chose this variable to denote a cycle as it was a reliable parameter in the files, clearly noted and described, since the files from 2000 were handwritten and, most importantly, not yet standardized. We did not include hormonal preparations on women—which, in other studies, are considered as starting an IVF cycle—that may have ended with no egg retrievals. (Therefore, the number of women who may have started with IVF treatment was higher than the number reported in this study.)

Treatments included egg retrievals and embryo transfers, fresh and frozen/thawed. The number of treatments (including egg retrieval and embryo transfers, fresh and frozen/thawed) in the 2000 cohort ranged from one to 25. The average number of treatments (not including previous treatments in other clinics) was 4.5 ($SD = 3.3$); around 10% of the women had more than eight treatments (22 women out of 210). The range of cycles (egg retrievals) in the 2000 cohort ranged from one to 22. The average number of cycles (including cycles in other clinics) was 4.0 ($SD = 3.1$); and 20.5% of the women had more than five cycles (43 women out of 210); 12.4% had more than seven cycles (26 women out of 210).

Rates of Live Births with IVF

In this study, success was defined as a live birth during one of the IVF cycles (unrelated to the order of pregnancy—either singleton or multiple—and the health status of the child). In the 2000 cohort, 86 women out of 210 succeeded in having a child with IVF (40.9%); however, more than half of the women (124 women out of 210) did not. Figure 8.1 presents the rate of success among the 2000 cohort by age at start of treatment. Among the women who started IVF before they turned 35, 49.2% succeeded in having a child (69 out of 141). In the over 35 age group, 20.9% of the women succeeded (25 women out of 68), and over the age of 40, less than one in 10 women succeeded with IVF (three women out of 32) (Fig. 8.1).

The rate of success was measured as the proportion of live births out of the overall number of IVF cycles. Out of 680 cycles in the 2000 cohort, the success rate was 21% (146 cycles). It is important to note here that we did not state the number of singletons, twins, and triplets, as the purpose of this study was to assess the number of IVF cycles ending in successful childbirth, not to count the overall number of children born. In addition, as mentioned above, we did not count women who started

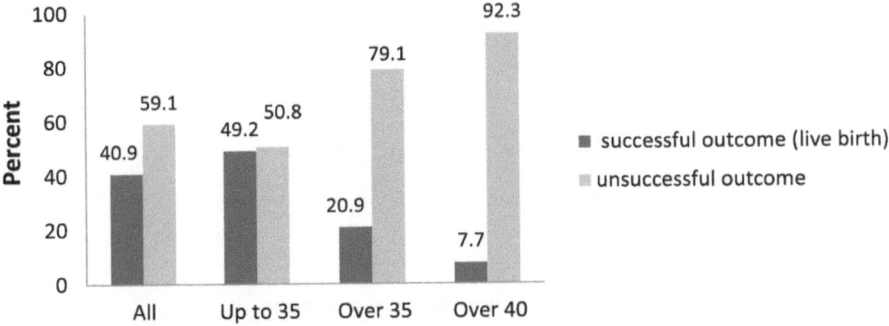

Fig. 8.1 Rate of success with IVF according to age at the start of treatment

hormonal treatment (usually considered as the start of an IVF cycle) but did not undergo egg retrieval.

Cumulative Rate of Live Births Over Time

Duration of infertility was relevant. Figure 8.2 presents the cumulative rates of success with a living birth over the years among the 2000 cohort. The line of cumulative rate of success was pronouncedly up in the first year (0.314 probability) and somewhat less pronounced but still up in the second year (an addition of 0.104 probability). However, the line becomes almost horizontal after the second year; that is, with no additional successful outcomes (or, with a rare miraculous event at some point).

We first presented this figure downwards for publication ("effect of time over rate of success with IVF"). The reviewers, however, did not approve our graph and demanded the figure be drawn upwards (thus "cumulative rate of success of IVF"),

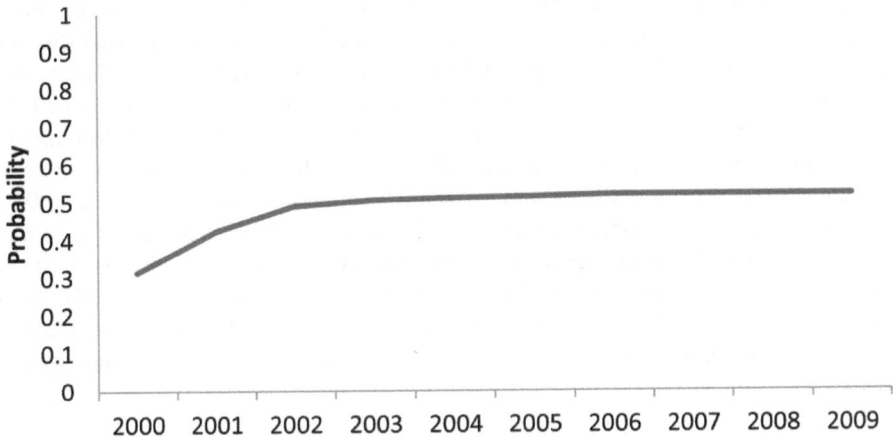

Fig. 8.2 Cumulative rate of live births over time

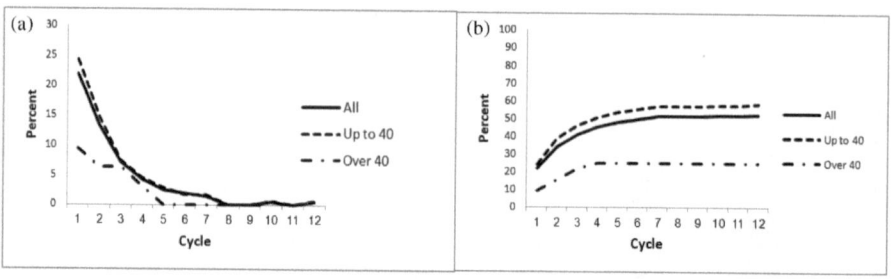

Fig. 8.3 Success rate by cycle and age at the start of IVF treatment

which we did. However, although drawing the figure upwards is legitimate, it is also misleading.[3] Indeed, when the figure goes up, the overall impression is that things will improve with the number of cycles. The truth is that the situation gets worse, i.e., the more years that go by and the more cycles a woman does, the probability of conceiving with IVF diminishes. Indeed, the flattening of the curve (i.e., zero deliveries) occurs also when the figure is drawn upwards. Many lay people may miss this crucial point.

Live Birth Rates by Cycle

Figure 8.3 presents the cumulative rates of success with a living birth among the women who started the treatment with IVF in 2000, by number of cycles and the age of the women at the start of treatment (under and over 40). Overall, among the 2000 cohort, 21.9% of the women succeeded in having a child in the first cycle (46 women out of 210), 13.3% of the women succeeded in the second cycle, 7.1% in the third cycle (15 women out of 210), and 4.3% in the fourth (nine women out of 210). In the fifth cycle, the probability of success plummeted to less than 3%. In the seventh cycle, the probability of success fell to less than 1%. Among the women who began IVF treatment over the age of 40, the rate of success after the fourth cycle was null.

We presented this figure downwards as well (Fig. 8.3a), but the journal did not approve it and demanded that the graph be drawn upwards. We complied (Fig. 8.3b). This notwithstanding, as the original (downward) chart clearly reveals, the more IVF cycles women underwent, the less successful they were at having a child. Among the 2000 cohort, there was a significant age difference at the start of treatment between women who succeeded with IVF and women who did not ($t(184) = 4.29, p < 0.001$). The average age of women who succeeded with IVF ($M = 30.7, SD = 5.2$) was significantly lower than the age of the women who did not succeed ($M = 34.3, SD = 6.6$). Moreover, contrary to the optimistic successful pattern in, Fig. 8.3b, Fig. 8.3a shows clearly how useless it is to go through more and more IVF cycles; a fact that the expert reviewers at Fertility and Sterility (and others) obviously do not want women to see (see also Chap. 7).

---

[3] For a compelling account about misleading statistics, see Darrel Huff's book: How To Lie With Statistics, London: Penguin (1991).

In Figs. 8.2 and 8.3b, we present the success percentage up to 100%, so the highest line appears in the middle of the chart. The Israeli Ministry of Health chart showing the success rate of live births through the years presents the success percentage only up to 35%.[6] Since the lines curve upwards and appear at the top of the figure (35%), lay people (and others) may assume that the overall success with IVF is high. Although cutting off part of the chart to focus on certain lines is not necessarily wrong, in the case of the IVF success rate, it is again misleading.

Physiological Data and Health Status

The patients' files in both IVF clinics did not contain complete physiological data, so we could not follow (possible) effect/s of the treatment with IVF on physiological parameters. However, 43% of the women in the 2000 cohort were hospitalized at least once during IVF treatments (90 out of 210 women). We did not test the reasons for hospitalization, because in most cases, they were not clearly stated in the file. Some patients' files recorded hospitalization due to early pregnancy complications following IVF-ET treatment for several reasons, such as abdominal pain or vaginal bleeding. These patients are considered at high risk for several pregnancy complications and their level of stress is always high. The number of hospitalizations per woman in this cohort ranged from zero to seven. The average number of hospitalizations was 0.84 ($SD = 1.4$). There was also a significant positive correlation (although weak) between the number of treatments and the number of hospitalizations ($r = 0.17, p < 0.01$); in other words, women who had undergone more IVF treatments had been hospitalized more times. Among women who did not succeed in having a child with IVF, this correlation was somewhat stronger ($r = 0.26, p < 0.01$).

In addition, we examined newer data from women who were in treatment with IVF in 2010 in order to evaluate whether there were some recognizable patterns. This group was not equal to the 2000 cohort since it included women who were still in either short- or long-term treatment; nevertheless, this group could offer some insights on developing trends in IVF clinics. Plausibly, in the group that was in treatment during 2010, younger women who may have succeeded in previous cycles were not included. Even so, the age at the start of treatment in this group was the same as at the start of treatment in 2000 ($M = 32.5$). Standard deviation was similar ($SD = 6.2$ and $SD = 6.3$ respectively), suggesting that age at the start of treatment with IVF may not have gone up since 2000. Nonetheless, the 2010 cohort included 12 women aged 18–22 compared with only three women of 20–22 in the 2000 cohort.

Moreover, the 2010 cohort included an 18-year-old (!) and a 19-year-old. We found no explanation in the files for why these very young women were undergoing IVF treatment. But the fourfold increase in a decade of very young women doing IVF (12 women in 2010 compared with three in 2000) suggests that more women may be aware of the declining success of IVF with age. It is also possible that women are overstressed about reproductive matters. As reproduction for Israeli women is viewed as a must and infertility is considered a terrible curse (see Chap. 3), women in Israel may rush into IVF at a younger age.

The WHO currently defines infertility as "the inability of a sexually active, non-contracepting couple to achieve pregnancy in one year,"[7] but this definition has changed over the years. Previously, infertility was defined as the inability to conceive after two years of unprotected intercourse. Plausibly, the definition changed because age in IVF does matter. This fact also seems to cause stress to women who want a baby (and their physicians). IVF in Israel may start after only six months of unprotected intercourse; some women may still give inaccurate data (i.e., tell a lie) about the length of time they had been trying to get pregnant (personal communication).

The number of treatments among the 2010 group (which at the time of the research were still ongoing) ranged between one and 21, the average number of treatments (not including treatments in other clinics) was 5.0 ($SD = 3.7$); and 14.5% of the women had already undergone more than eight treatments (47 women out of 325). The number of cycles (egg retrievals) in this group ranged from one to 20. Average number of cycles (including reported cycles in other clinics) was 4.1 ($SD = 3.1$). In addition, 25.2% of the women had already undergone more than five cycles (82 women out of 325), 12.3% of the women in 2010 had already done more than seven cycles (40 women out of 325). During 2010 alone, there were 459 cycles and 76 live births. Thus, the rate of success with IVF during 2010 in this study was 16.6%, higher than the official national success rate in 2010 (which was 14.9%).

As in the 2000 cohort, age in 2010 remained relevant for a successful outcome. Although we could not capture the whole picture (younger women who may have succeeded in previous treatments), there was still a significant difference in the average age at the start of treatment between women who had succeeded with IVF— at the time we had looked at the records—and women who had not ($t(309) = 6.57, p < 0.001$). The average age among women who succeeded with IVF during 2010 ($M = 30.0, SD = 5.3$) was significantly lower than the average age among those who did not succeed ($M = 34.3, SD = 6.3$).

Discussion

We gathered retrospective data from 535 files in two IVF clinics, from patients who began IVF treatment in 2000 (n = 210) and patients who were in IVF treatment during 2010 (n = 325). Less than half of the 2000 cohort succeeded with IVF treatment (41%), which means that many families did produce a child with the aid of IVF. However, more than half of the women in the 2000 cohort were unsuccessful. In this study, 26% of the women in the clinics that we reviewed had previously undergone IVF in another clinic. The fact that almost two thirds of these patients entered these two clinics between the first and the third cycle may indicate that these specific IVF centers may have a better reputation than others.

In this study, the overall IVF success rate in both clinics during 2010 was 16.6%; higher than the official IVF success rate during 2010 in Israel of just 14.9%.[8] We acknowledge the limitation that we did not trace women who might have continued treatment in another clinic. (At the time of writing, a national follow up of women who may move from one clinic to another remains unavailable.) Nevertheless, in this study, with each new cycle, the rate of success with IVF diminished. Even if we look at the figure in the upward direction, we can see that over seven cycles with IVF, the rate of success was almost zero; and this included the women who had undergone previous cycles in other IVF clinics. In addition, we calculated the cumulative pregnancy rate per year in the 2000 cohort. If we look at the figure in the upward direction, we see an escalating line during the first two years. Further along, the line becomes a plateau, indicating no more successful pregnancies, but this happens long before women may give up. This pattern suggests that a "culture of perseverance" with IVF cycles is at work in Israeli clinics. Certainly, one of the reasons for this pattern is the policy of unlimited IVF in Israel. Nonetheless, a cumulative figure, which is inherently positive, is highly relevant in this discussion, as lay people may misrepresent the cumulative rates of a successful outcome. Indeed, lay people may think that the escalating line does mean "keep going and you will succeed," but this is not the case with IVF treatment. Still, this belief seems to be at the core of the limitless policy for IVF in Israel.

According to Selah et al. (2013) there were fewer successes with IVF in Israel in the years 2007–2009. They suggested that this decline was due to treatments with IVF when the chances of success were poor in the first place. In our study, the rate of women who had already undergone more than seven cycles in 2010 was 12%, the same rate of women who underwent more than seven cycles in the 2000 cohort (Simonstein et al. 2014). However, as the group of 2010 had not yet finished with IVF treatment, it is likely that the number of IVF cycles—with poorer chances of success—continued to climb in the years following our research.

Higher rates of hospitalizations with multi cycles are noteworthy; moreover, a stronger correlation was found between multi cycles and higher rates of hospitalization among women who did not succeed in having a child. While these data remain at the exploratory level, with the lack of availability of further details on hospitalization to shed light on the patients' clinical situation, the controversy continues regarding possible negative effects resulting from hormonal treatment (Brinton et al. 2005; Calderon-Margalit et al. 2009; Jensen et al. 2008), which remain uncertain. Weirdly, a study carried out by the Research Department of the Israeli Knesset that reviewed the data published about women diagnosed with cancer following IVF treatment concluded that the studies suggesting that fertility hormones may cause cancer are "irrelevant" in IVF because women doing IVF receive higher doses of hormones (!?) (Dror 2005). A newer version of this report suggests the opposite, i.e., that women in IVF take fewer hormones, and therefore the studies relating to reproductive hormones remain "irrelevant" (again) to the Israeli case.[9] In both these reports, IVF remains spotless.

We suggested in this study that further examination of hospitalizations, both during and after IVF treatment, is necessary (Simonstein et al. 2014). At the time of writing this chapter in August 2020, this has not been performed. What has happened, however, is that in 2014, the Israeli Ministry of Health drafted a new guideline concerning the number of cycles with IVF.

8.3   The 2014 Guideline for IVF in Israel[(10)]

The new directions state that women aged up to 39 may undergo IVF treatments based on medical considerations as "*a first option;*" women aged up to 42 will not undergo more than three consecutive IVF treatments in which they did not reach the embryo returning stage during treatment. Nevertheless, if embryos were returned, even in the third cycle, "the count starts again." Finally, the guidelines state that at any age, after four consecutive months of treatment, in which they did not reach the embryo returning stage, or after eight IVF cycles, the attending team will conduct "a discussion at the responsibility of the unit in which the last treatment cycle was performed." This discussion will concern "the reasons for the failure and suggestions for further treatment." The plan for further treatment "including additional IVF treatments" will be determined "according to the conclusions of the discussion."[(11)]

These guidelines seem reasonable, taking into account the ineffectiveness of IVF treatment after a certain age and after many cycles. However, the document is not binding. The wording of the guideline is permissive, leaving the decision of whether to continue with IVF up to the IVF unit. Moreover, while a couple's infertility can result from either the man or the woman, and can sometimes be easily resolved if it is the man's problem, it is almost always the woman who endures the infertility treatment (personal communication). Based on the belief that a woman without a child is "incomplete" as she has not reached her goal as a woman, it is argued that "no one can stop a woman pursuing her wish for a baby" and therefore "no one can decide to stop a woman's IVF treatment if she wants to continue" (personal communication).[4] And women do continue. Indeed, a study carried out in 2010, by sociologist Remennick from Bar Ilan University, observed that some women reported being in IVF treatment for around seven years (Remennick 2000). Translated into cycles of IVF, this means that a woman in Israel may undergo between 35 and 42 cycles.

Should There Be A(ny) Limit to IVF Cycles?

It has been noted in the international discussion of assistive reproductive technology that funding mechanisms for IVF should maximize efficiency and equity of access while minimizing the potential harm from multiple births (Chambers et al. 2009). However, many other potential harms and risks of IVF have been ignored, overlooked, and/or not yet addressed. While many view the Israeli policy as optimal, the implications of a policy of unlimited rounds of IVF from the perspective of the "culture of perseverance" that develops in IVF clinics has not yet been fully assessed—either in Israel or elsewhere (Simonstein 2010). Age remains a major factor; the odds are better for younger women and deteriorate with age. The number of unsuccessful cycles of IVF is also predictive of a negative outcome, which is inconsistent with the Israeli policy of unlimited rounds.

---

[4] Even age has remained open to question, as I witnessed a counseling session in which the woman's date of birth was manipulated.

The number of IVF cycles that a woman in Israel may undergo remains unknown. In 2010, the number of IVF cycles had doubled compared with the number in 2000. By 2017—the last report available at the time of writing (August 2020)—the number of IVF cycles compared with 2000 had almost tripled. Yet, over the last two decades, the success rate per IVF cycle in Israel has remained constant at 15–17%. Whereas 20% may be the natural rate of conception after unprotected intercourse,[5] the natural process may be enjoyable and does not compromise the woman's health. By contrast, IVF is a demanding medical procedure, costly in time and money, but primarily demands physical and psychological investment by the woman.

8.4 Discussion Revisited

The claim in favor of the huge investment required of women for IVF is that women invest in a pregnancy in any case. Indeed, pregnancy and birth has always been a dangerous process for women. Enhanced healthcare has greatly improved the situation, but women still die from reproductive hazards, before, during, or after labor. The World Health Organization estimates that more than 300,000 women died from pregnancy-related causes in 2015—i.e., 830 women every day.[1] Most of these pregnancy-related deaths occur in developing countries, but even in the United States, about 700 women die each year as a result of either pregnancy or delivery complications.[12]

IVF, requiring first the injection of hormones, and then general anesthesia during egg retrieval, adds to the perils of a natural pregnancy. Despite reports of increased risk of some forms of cancer due to IVF, the policy of unlimited cycles of IVF in Israel has never been put on hold. The risks have not been assimilated by the public, the health system, or the Knesset. Although most women submit themselves to IVF unquestioningly, grateful that it might "cure" their infertility status, the effectiveness of the almost open-ended IVF policy in Israel remains unclear. Media reports of successes after many years in IVF are rare. Paradoxically, while these rare successes are regarded as miraculous events (their very newsworthiness testifies to this), they do mislead people's beliefs regarding success with IVF. The upward figures produced by the IVF experts do the rest. Many people believe that IVF success is very high and that the key to success is perseverance. Nonetheless, the public's present perception of higher pregnancy rates with IVF is unfounded.

According to Remennick (2000), many Israeli women may find themselves worse off after many years of IVF: still without a child, but also disfigured (overweight because of the hormonal injections), their partnerships lost (because of the stress and

---

[5] According to Marantz-Henig in Pandora's Baby, 20% probability of natural conception per month can be found also on the Women's Reproductive Center website: https://womensreproduction.com/what-are-normal-conception-rates/ and on a website dealing with health matters: https://www.health.com/condition/pregnancy/pregnancy-odds-fertility-success-rates-in-your-30s-and-40s. The Medical News Today website states that the rate of natural conception per month is 30%. https://www.medicalnewstoday.com/articles/chances-of-getting-pregnant-first-time-trying.

lack of sexual intimacy), and their careers ruined (through time spent feeling sick) because of the treatment. Women who did not succeed in having a baby after many years of IVF explain that the support for women's right to become mothers in Israel encourages women to keep on trying to become pregnant. As having children is a "moral duty" for women in Israel (but not only in Israel),[6] they feel that they cannot possibly avoid the technology. Moreover, in Israel, it is illegal to dismiss a woman from her job because she is undergoing IVF treatment. So, women say that since the State provides IVF free of charge,[13] they feel an "obligation" not to discontinue treatment. Thus, under such "ideal" conditions, if a woman finally decides to stop treatment, she must shoulder the blame for the failure (Remennick 2000).

Is IVF an Ongoing Experiment?

By 2018, 8 million of children had been born through IVF,[14] which has become "routine." Indeed, according to Niederberger and Pellicer, the chief editors of the Fertility and Sterility journal, and the editors of the special issue of the journal celebrating 40 years of IVF, the rate of implantation had improved tenfold during that time, from 5 to 50% (Niederberger and Pellicer 2018). They observed, however, that:

> The low implantation rates of the early days was *problematically addressed* by increasing the number of embryos replaced into the uterus and *aggressive ovarian stimulation protocols, unfortunately often uncontrolled*, introducing the two main complications of IVF in these 40 years—multiple pregnancies and ovarian hyper stimulation syndrome (OHS). (Niederberger and Pellicer 2018, p. 188) [my italics]

Uteruses and ovaries are female organs but, interestingly, women are not mentioned. The phraseology used in relation to these organs is completely reminiscent of experimentation; in other words, experimenting with women. In the opinion of Niederberger and Pellicer, the challenges have been "almost completely resolved;" but according to the CDC, there were 68,908 live births in 2018 (24.2% success) but 78,052 live born infants, meaning that there were still 9144 multiple pregnancies.[15] Moreover, OHS remains underreported. A hospitalization following IVF treatment is considered as "pregnancy complications" and not necessarily due to the IVF procedure (personal communication).

Niederberger and Pellicer (2018) observe also that the protocols of controlled ovarian hyperstimulation (COH) have undergone "substantial evolution," mainly due to the research and development of "new therapeutic agents." It is true that reproductive hormones are now produced in the laboratory. Pergonal, a drug used for many years in IVF, was obtained from the urine of postmenstrual women, containing the gonadotropic hormones (FSH and LH) that are necessary for IVF treatment. However, this drug contained other compounds present in the urine, not only the relevant hormones for ovarian stimulation. The result was side effects, ranging from mild to serious, for the women receiving the medication.

---

[6] A max reasserted recently by the Pope; but particularly in Israel, a pronatalist country (see Chaps. 3 and 4).

The journal editors acknowledge that they "have learned" over time: for example, they explain that "overly aggressive management of the ovaries was detrimental to a woman's reproductive system." Learning here means experimenting. This begs the question of how many women received this "overly aggressive" treatment. The answer remains unknown. According to the editors, current management of COH is "completely different" from 40 years ago (Niederberger and Pellicer 2018). The hormones that are currently injected in IVF to a woman's body are synthetic and, therefore, cleaner. Today, however, it is well known that women respond differently to the stimulation compound. Thus, protocols may have improved, but each woman starting with IVF, in fact, becomes a new experiment.

8.5 Conclusions

The Israeli policy of IVF may be considered by many as very generous, and as consistent with women's "needs" and "rights." At first sight, the Israeli policy might be taken as an example to be followed worldwide as it seems to be a win–win situation, with all the stakeholders benefiting equally under the ultra-permissive policy. However, a closer examination suggests that this may not be the case. Israeli women embark on very lengthy IVF treatment, ending up worse off in too many cases. Low-cost treatment with IVF may help some women but may become a "perseverance trap" for others. Indeed, the "culture of perseverance" with IVF in Israel has been on the rise—against the odds and despite other health hazards.

The effectiveness of an open-ended IVF policy is problematic, but in Israel—even with a cautionary but quite ineffectual guideline—this policy has remained in place. Moreover, the low efficacy of any single IVF cycle remains questionable. Although IVF is now considered routine, the procedure remains highly ineffective as fewer than half the women will actually take a baby home; and each cycle with IVF has an average of 83–85% failure. In addition, the side effects of long-term treatment with IVF have remained unclear.

During (and before) the 1970s, IVF began as an experiment on childless women (see Chap. 7). Sometimes, even without their knowledge, they were in fact human guinea pigs. Nowadays, women sign an informed consent form, but it remains questionable how really informed women are, as misleading information about IVF has generally got the upper hand. In fact, the informed consent document is formulated to give full protection from any charges to the clinic and its physicians.

In the context of womb politics, we may assume that not many (or not any?) men would submit themselves to a non-life-saving, demanding, and risky medical procedure, with more than 80% rate of failure per cycle [!] that has now remained constant for two decades. Nevertheless, IVF's Teflon reputation still stands. IVF has become the primary route to treat infertility and is a thriving industry worldwide—and certainly in Israel. In our study, we recommended a systematic long-term assessment of the health and welfare of the women after IVF—especially after prolonged treatment; and suggested that further *independent* research, both retrospective and prospective, is needed to develop a truly informed policy for IVF in Israel and worldwide, which could assist patients' (women's) needs and also protect their health.[7]

In the not too distant future, however, as we will see in the next chapter, all women—not only women experiencing infertility—may find themselves facing further reproductive risks and experimentation with the development of reprogenetics.

Notes

(1)   https://ourworldindata.org/how-many-women-die-in-childbirth. Accessed 1 Aug 2020.
(2)   In vitro fertilization (IVF) treatments 1990–2017. Report October 2019. https://www.health. gov.il/PublicationsFiles/IVF1990-2017.pdf. Accessed 27 July 2020.
(3)   NHI website. http://www.health.gov.il. Accessed 2 Oct 2010.
(4)   Data based on: CBS, Population Census; Population and immigration authority, Population Register. https://old.cbs.gov.il/reader/cw_usr_view_SHTML?ID=803. Accessed 22 July 2020.
(5)   https://www.health.gov.il/Subjects/Med_Inst/IVF/Pages/IVF-list.aspx. Accessed 5 Aug 2020.
(6)   https://www.health.gov.il/PublicationsFiles/IVF1990-2018.pdf. Accessed 25 Aug 2020.
(7)   https://www.who.int/reproductivehealth/topics/infertility/definitions/en/. Accessed 30 July 2020.
(8)   Israel Health ministry website (3 Sept 2013). http://www.health.gov.il/PublicationsFiles/IVF 1986_2010.pdf.
(9)   https://fs.knesset.gov.il/globaldocs/MMM/f168cce7-8e32-e811-80de-00155d0a0235/2_f 168cce7-8e32-e811-80de-00155d0a0235_11_10167.pdf. Accessed 1 Aug 2020.
(10)   https://www.health.gov.il/hozer/mr06_2014.pdf (Hebrew). Accessed 1 Aug 2020.
(11)   https://www.health.gov.il/English/Topics/fertility/Pages/ivf.aspx. Accessed 1 Aug 2020.
(12)   https://www.cdc.gov/reproductivehealth/maternalinfanthealth/pregnancy-relatedmortality. htm. Accessed 1 Aug 2020.
(13)   https://www.health.gov.il/PublicationsFiles/English/IVF-handbook_EN.pdf. Accessed 5 Aug 2020.
(14)   https://www.sciencedaily.com/releases/2018/07/180703084127.htm. Accessed 3 Aug 2020.
(15)   https://www.cdc.gov/art/artdata/index.html. Accessed 3 Aug 2020.

References

Aksoy, S. 2004. Response to: A Rational Cure for Pre-Reproductive Stress Syndrome. *Journal of Medical Ethics* 30: 382–383.

---

[7] While the equitable nature of access to IVF in Israel should be applauded, in the context of NHI constraints, a scheme of (almost) limitless rounds of IVF remains questionable. A scheme of limitless rounds of IVF should be weighed (transparently) against other health care needs. In a global context, an evidence-based policy on assistive reproductive technologies may improve both the allocation of resources and the duty of care, not only in Israel, but also in other countries.

Bennet, R. 2004. Human Reproduction: Irrational But in Most Cases Morally Defensible. *Journal of Medical Ethics* 30: 379–380.

Brinton, L.A., K.S. Moghissi, B. Scoccia, C.L. Westhoff, and E.J. Lamb. 2005. Ovulation Induction and Cancer Risk. *Fertility and Sterility* 83: 261–274.

Calderon-Margalit, R., Y. Friedlander, R. Yanetz, K. Kleinhaus, M.C. Perrin, O. Manor, et al. 2009. Cancer Risk After Exposure to Treatments for Ovulation Induction. *American Journal of Epidemiology* 169: 365–375.

Chambers, G.M., E.A. Sullivan, O. Ishihara, et al. 2009. The Economic Impact of Assisted Reproductive Technology: A Review of Selected Developed Countries. *Fertility and Sterility* 91: 2281–2294.

Cook, R., B.M. Dickens, and M.F. Fathalla. 2003. *Reproductive Health and Human Rights*, 29. New York: Oxford University Press.

Damianov, L. 2002. *A Possibility to Prevent the Catastrophe*. Bulgarian Association of Sterility & Reproductive Health (in Bulgarian). http://www.zachatie.org/index.php?option=com_content&task=view&id=456&Itemid=30. Accessed 5 Mar 2010.

Dror, T. 2005. *Breast Cancer and Other Risks in Assisted Reproduction*. Data and Research Center of the Knesset (in Hebrew). Available at http://www.knesset.gov.il/MMM/data/pdf/m01213.pdf. Accessed 17 Sept 2010.

Henig, M.R. 2004. *Pandora's Baby*. New York: Houghton Mifflin.

Häyry, M. 2004. A Rational Cure for Pre-Reproductive Stress Syndrome. *Journal of Medical Ethics* 30: 377–378.

Holm, S. 2004. Why It Is Not Strongly Irrational to Have Children. *Journal of Medical Ethics* 30: 381.

Holm, Soren. 2009. The Medicalisation of Reproduction—A 30 Years Perspective. In *Reprogen-Ethics and the Future of Gender*, ed. Frida Simonstein, 29–36. London: Springer.

Jensen, A., H. Sharif, J.H. Olsen, and S.K. Kjaer. 2008. Risk of Breast Cancer and Gynecologic Cancers in a Large Population of Nearly 50,000 Infertile Danish Women. *American Journal of Epidemiology* 168: 49–57.

Malizia, B., M.R. Hacker, and A.S. Penzias. 2009. Cumulative Live-Birth Rates After In Vitro Fertilization. *New England Journal of Medicine* 360: 236–243.

Nachtigall, R.D. 2006. International Disparities in Access to Infertility Services. *Fertility and Sterility* 85: 871–875.

Niederberger, C., and A. Pellicer. 2018. Introduction. Forty Years of IVF. *Fertility and Sterility* 110 (2): 188–310. https://doi.org/10.1016/j.fertnstert.2018.06.005.

Pelinck, M.J., H.M. Knol, N.E.A. Vogel, E.G.J.M. Arts, A.H.M. Simons, et al. 2008. Cumulative Pregnancy Rates After Sequential Treatment with Modified Natural Cycle IVF Followed by IVF with Controlled Ovarian Stimulation. *Human Reproduction* 23: 1808–1814.

Remennick, L. 2000. Childless in the Land of Imperative Motherhood: Stigma and Coping Among Infertile Israeli Women. *Sex Roles* 43: 821–841.

Selah, T., I. Segal, A. Goran, G. Hudik, V. Shalev, H. Homberg, et al. 2013. In Vitro Fertilization at Macabbi Health Care Services 2007–2010. *Harefuah* 52: 11–15 (Hebrew).

Simonstein, F. 2010. Assisted Reproduction Policies with Emphasis on Israeli Practices. *Health Policy* 97: 202–208.

Simonstein, F., and E. Balabanova. 2009. 'Can't Avoid It, Can't Afford It': Assisted Reproduction in Israel and Bulgaria. In *Reprogen-Ethics and the Future of Gender*, ed. F. Simonstein, 55–64. London: Springer.

Simonstein, F., and M. Mashiach-Eizenberg. 2012. How Long Should Women Persevere with IVF? *Journal of Health Services Research & Policy* 17 (2): 121–123.

Simonstein, F., M. Mashiach-Eizenberg, A. Revel, and J.S. Younis. 2014. Assisted Reproduction Policies in Israel: A Retrospective Analysis of In Vitro Fertilization–Embryo Transfer. *Fertility and Sterility* 102 (5): 1301–1306.

Younis, J.S., O. Radin, N. Mirsky, I. Izhaki, T. Majara, et al. 2008. First Polar Body and Nucleolar Precursor Body Morphology Is Related to the Ovarian Reserve of Infertile Women. *Reproductive Biomedicine Online* 16: 851–858.

Younis, J.S., M. Ben-Ami, I. Izhaki, J. Jadaon, B. Brenner, and G. Sarig. 2013. The Association Between Poor Ovarian Response and Thrombophilia in Assisted Reproduction. *European Journal of Obstetrics, Gynecology, and Reproductive Biology* 166: 65–69.

Chapter 9
Reprogenetics

The word reprogenetics combines assisted reproduction and molecular genetics, namely in vitro fertilization (IVF) and gene editing. The word was first coined in 1998 in the book Remaking Eden—soon after the birth of Dolly the sheep—by geneticist Lee Silver (1998). Silver foresaw the merging of two separate sciences: molecular genetics (i.e., gene editing) and assisted reproduction (i.e., IVF).[1] Since then, there has been a continuous race to improve gene editing tools. At the time of writing, CrisprQCas9 remains a highly efficient and much less expensive technique than those previously used to target genes (Ran et al. 2013; Senior 2015).

While I was on a sabbatical in London, an article on the front page of The Independent, in September 2015, reported that the "genetic manipulation of IVF embryos" was to start in Britain, using "a new revolutionary gene-editing technique, called Crispr/Cas9." About three weeks later, in October 2015, it was reported on the front page of the same newspaper that the National Health Service (NHS) had faced a 1 billion pound deficit only three months into the New Year. The chief executive of Monitor remarked that overspending on this scale could not be attributed to either mismanagement or waste amongst individual trusts, but reflected "the impossible task" of delivering high-quality care to patients due to inadequate funding. The hidden connection between these two reports was that gene editing with CrispR/Cas—or any other enzymatic tool if proved safe—could be used to solve issues related to health care allocation. Reprogenetics involving gene editing could improve people's health, resulting, by and large, in substantial betterment to public health. Indeed, according to Bostrom and Savulescu (2013 [2009]), advances in the biomedical sciences suggest that it will become "increasingly feasible" to use medicine and technology "to enhance basic human capacities," including controlling the biological processes underlying normal aging (Bostrom and Savulescu 2013 [2009]).

---

[1] Silver noted that through genetic enhancing, two species of humans will develop: those who were genetically enhanced and those who were not. Since enhancing would require monetary investment, enhanced people would not want to waste their "better" gene pool by mating with non-enhanced people. See Silver's *Enhancing Humans*.

© The Author(s), under exclusive license to Springer Nature Switzerland AG 2022   129
F. Simonstein, *Womb Politics: A Short History of the Future of Human Reproduction*,
The International Library of Bioethics 99,
https://doi.org/10.1007/978-3-031-11654-4_8

Enhancing future generations, however, will require IVF and preimplantation genetic diagnosis (PGD). This evidently requires the involvement of women in the process, but remarkably, women's necessary involvement in an enhancing scenario has not been discussed by its proponents (Bostrom and Savulescu 2013 [2009]; Harris 2013 [2009]; Savulescu 2006; Savulescu et al. 2015). Moreover, the present discourse on moral obligations of future generations, although not referring to women, seems to imply that women might be required morally, if not legally, to reproduce with IVF. This chapter focuses on health care allocation related to gene editing and the possibility of enhancing future generations. It examines the crucial involvement of women in a scenario of enhancing reproduction and looks at the artificial womb (AW) as a means of ensuring women's autonomy and choice.

9.1   Health Care Allocation

Starting from the second half of the twentieth century, humans have been exceptionally good at avoiding the risk of premature death, mostly of newborns and children, but also of adolescents and adults. During the last century, life expectancy at birth in developed countries increased by more than 30 years, which is a formidable achievement of science and medicine. Paradoxically, however, humans now live long enough to become stricken with late onset, chronic diseases. Illnesses have now shifted from "acute" to "chronic" (The EU Summit on Chronic Diseases 2014). Common, general, and chronic diseases such as high blood pressure, diabetes, osteoporosis, hypercholesterolemia, kidney failure, heart disease, Alzheimer's and Parkinson's are manifesting themselves as people live longer. As society ages, more people need health care, including long-term care.

The 2020 COVID-19 pandemic has badly affected older people and those with chronic illnesses. At the time of writing, there is no cure, but successful vaccines have been developed. They will help to contain COVID-19 until it eventually disappears, as happened with many other pandemics, either with a vaccine, e.g., smallpox, or without, e.g., the Spanish flu. The trouble is that, even once COVID-19 is controlled or destroyed, chronic diseases will remain. Some experts have suggested that long-term care might be the major health and social issue of the next four decades, polarizing society over the next 20–40 years. In this context, there is a growing discussion about the need to ration medical treatment that is considered beneficial. Many writers suggest that societies should worry about such trends and must reassess cultural and social norms (Walker 2009; Zimmer and McDaniel 2013). Enhancing the health of future people by gene editing might, one day, become a morally preferable solution to rationing medical treatment.

9.2 Gene Editing

Gene editing involves making a change in the genetic material (the C, G, A, Ts) of the organism in question. A specific sequence of this genetic material is a code that generates a particular protein in the body. Proteins are large, complex molecules that play critical roles in the body. They are required for the structure, function, and regulation of the body's tissues and organs and do most of the work in cells. A genetic modification refers to a change made in the genetic code, by inserting either new genetic material or a gene, by knocking down a gene, or by activating or inactivating a gene. The new tool for editing genes with Crispr/Cas9 might further improve the results of gene editing, since the new technique is cheaper and easier to handle than other, existing techniques.

The act of gene editing may target somatic cells (i.e., all the cells in the body excluding the reproductive cells) or the cells in the "germline" (i.e., the reproductive cells that might develop in a new organism). Gene editing of somatic cells to cure disease is considered acceptable, and has been tried with mixed results. However, targeting the germline in humans has, so far, remained forbidden. At present, at least 25 countries worldwide have banned human germ cell modification, including 15 EU nations, Canada, Brazil, Mexico, and Australia. Laws in Germany and Austria are particularly restrictive (Senior 2015). The American government has imposed a moratorium on federally funded research on embryos in the United States (go.nature.com/mgscb2). In Israel, a small but leading country in embryonic stem cell research, research on embryos has been permitted for medical research since 1999, but not for reproductive purposes (Simonstein 2008a). Germline gene therapy is illegal also in the United Kingdom; however, the IVF legislation was changed in 2008 to allow genetic interventions with human embryos for research purposes, but only if done under license (http://www.hfea.gov.uk/).

In February 2016, the Human Fertilization and Embryology Authority (HFEA) approved a request by the Francis Crick Institute in London to modify human embryos using the new gene editing technique CRISPR-Cas9 (http://www.hfea.gov.uk/). This was the second time human embryos were employed in such research, and the first time their use was allowed in the UK by a national regulatory authority. The embryos provided by patients undergoing IVF were not allowed to develop beyond seven days (http://www.hfea.gov.uk/). Nonetheless, in February 2018, Chinese scientists reported, for the first time, that they had used Crispr/Cas9 to alter "spare" human embryos genetically (Wang et al. 2015). Jiankui, a genome-editing researcher at the Southern University of Science and Technology of China in Shenzhen, claimed that he had edited the genomes of these first babies—twin girls—to make them resistant to HIV.[1] The report in Nature journal stated that by engineering mutations into human embryos, implanted in a woman's womb and brought to term, these Chinese scientists had, in fact, "started an era in which science could rewrite the gene pool of future generations by altering the human germline." According to the same report, Jiankui also ignored established norms for human safety and protection along the way; which "caused a general outcry as efforts to make heritable changes to the human genome are presently fraught with uncertainty."[2] Jiankui was dismissed from the University[1] and was later sentenced to three years in jail by a closed court in Shenzhen. He and two research colleagues were found "guilty of illegal medical practice by knowingly violating the country's regulations and ethical principles with their experiments."[3] (XinhuaNet 2019). Indeed, opponents of gene editing of the germline say that modifying human embryos is dangerous and unnatural and does not take into account the consent of future generations.

9.3 Genetic Enhancement

It may take some time until gene editing of the germline becomes safe and acceptable. Nevertheless, genetic enhancement of the germline is already in use, in PGD performed on IVF embryos to avoid a disease in the offspring. If we choose to implant an embryo that is free of disease instead of an embryo that might have the disease, we have already improved the germline. To date, PGD has been performed to avoid terrible inborn gene related diseases that are potentially deadly in childhood, e.g., Tay-Sachs, or diseases that might be difficult to manage and could be deadly in adolescence, such as cystic fibrosis and thalassemias. However, PGD has also been used to avoid early deaths in adulthood, for example, from familial breast cancer.

Progress in avoiding inborn genetic diseases can probably be made merely by selecting healthy embryos in a Petri dish, without actively intervening in the genetic makeup of the child. Yet, supposing that gene editing becomes safe—which is not currently the case—it might certainly improve public health, since the population will be healthier; individuals could enjoy better health during maturity and in the aging process, which might in turn benefit the whole community. Thus, genetic enhancement might be applicable for the public good, for example, when considering the acute global health crisis caused by COVID-19, to make people resistant to deadly viruses.

It could be argued, however, that vaccines can be developed to solve the problem of diseases caused by viruses. This renders genetic enhancement unnecessary against horizontally transmitted diseases that pass from one person to another. Nonetheless, there is the overwhelming prospect of chronic illnesses in adulthood—late-onset genetic diseases—passing vertically from one generation to the next, and a growing aging population in ill health because of chronic and degenerative diseases. Even before the COVID-19 pandemic in 2020, these phenomena were a cause of hospital overcrowding, which in turn results in failing health care systems. In this case, genetic enhancement of the germline could be sought to resolve these problems. In that event, women might be required to reproduce with IVF for the sake of the "public good." Presently, the selection of healthy embryos for implantation with PGD already involves women reproducing by IVF, but these women constitute a relatively small group. Enhancing future generations by editing the germline might require that *all* women reproduce using IVF.[2]

Genetic enhancement is clearly in sight. Indeed, according to Bostrom and Savulescu, the idea of genetic enhancement of humans moved, during the first decade of the twenty-first century, "from the realm of science fiction to that of practical ethics." (Bostrom and Savulescu 2013 [2009]). Harris foresaw this development back in the early 1990s, while discussing the ethics of genetic enhancement in his book, Wonderwoman and Superman (Harris 1993). My own research for the Ph.D. degree at the University of Manchester, in the UK (1999–2003), also focused on the ethics of genetic enhancement (Simonstein 2014). Furthermore, in the collaborative book, Human Enhancement, editors Savulesco and Bostrom observe that the rapid advances taking place in the biomedical sciences and related technological areas "make it clear that [genetic] human enhancing will become possible over the coming years or decades." In their view, the question has shifted from "is it science fiction?" to "should we do it?" Bostrom and Savulescu perceive the book as attempting to analyze what exactly "it" is referring to (Bostrom and Savulescu 2013 [2009], p. 18). In the book, 20 renowned bioethicists authored 18 chapters dealing with the many pros and cons of enhancing humans.[3] Not one of them, however, even mentioned the fact that, for genetic enhancement of future generations, women would have to conceive via IVF. I made no mention of this, either, in my Ph.D. research on human enhancing and bioethics. On completion of the ninth and final chapter of my Ph.D., I told John Harris, my advisor, that a tenth chapter should be written about the involvement of women in gene enhancement. Harris did not understand why. At that moment, the idea for this book was conceived.

"Easy PGD ?"

During the last years of the twentieth century, a renowned Israeli geneticist told me that embracing emerging genetic technologies is "inevitable" (personal communication). As a geneticist myself, I was surprised by her certainty. Two decades later, Henry T. Greely writes in *The End of Sex*, that pre-implantation diagnosis (PGD) is "inevitable."(Greely 2016). According to Greely, pre-implantation tests (PGT) will become "easy." By "easy," Greely refers to the developing PGD technologies, i.e., PGD that may still involve IVF, but would not require the maturation of eggs in a woman's body. For example, embryos could be obtained from embryonic stem cells and Yamanaka Factors[4] could be used to reverse normal tissue cells back to the stage of gametes. Another way would be to take immature eggs from an ovarian slice and mature the eggs in vitro. This procedure, Greely writes, would still require an operation, but women would not have to take hormones to mature eggs in vivo.

---

[2] A vivid example of such a scenario can be seen in the 1997 film GATTACA. But the film does not focus on all women necessarily reproducing only through IVF. The focus in the film is—as usual—only on the potential effects of enhancing regarding "optimal"—and sub-optimal—future generations.

[3] Among these writers there was only one woman.

[4] Yamanaka factors can reverse the behavior of a mature cell into its embryonic pluripotent state (ePSc). Shinya Yamanaka received the 2012 Nobel Prize in physiology for this discovery.

Greely discusses "easy PGD" from (almost) every perspective. How "easy PGD" may influence the embryo, the family, medicine, society, and legal matters; from legislature prohibiting "easy PGD" to legislature fully accepting it. He includes the freedom of states (and countries) regarding this decision and even medical tourism as a result of it. He even discusses how the genetic makeup of embryos could be changed using CRISPR/Cas technology. However, while "easy PGD" by Greely will create a situation in which, in order to have children, all women will need to have IVF, again, absent from his discussion—equaling the other important writers above and below—is the woman's perspective.

Indeed, "easy" PGD is not being developed to make women's reproductive lives—with PGD—easier. Easy PGD is developing to make PGD easier.

9.4 The Involvement of Women in Gene Enhancement

Would women have the choice of whether or not to participate in an enhancing scenario? Would it become an obligation? Would it be a moral duty and/or a legally binding scheme? Women do not appear at all in the debates and discussions about enhancing. Well-known advocates of enhancing (Bostrom and Savulescu 2013 [2009]; Harris 2013 [2009]; Savulescu 2006; Savulescu et al. 2015) and many others have never mentioned the role of women in this scenario. Might this be an indication that the proponents of an enhancing scenario regard women's engagement with IVF as obvious, and therefore, as taken for granted?

The discussion about enhancing the germline has focused only on future generations. Proponents of enhancement focus on creating "better" offspring, disease-free and resistant to other maladies (such as UV rays and aging), and fitter overall. In 2001, Savulescu introduced the principle of procreative beneficence (PPB), stating that parents have the obligation "to choose the child that is expected to have the best life." (Savulescu 2001, p. 10). Opponents of enhancement say that modifying human embryos is dangerous and unnatural, and does not take the consent of future generations into account. Opponents of enhancement focus mainly on making taller and blonder "better looking" people. For example, Darnovsky, executive director of the Center for Genetics and Society, writes as follows:

> From a policy perspective, how would we draw the distinction between a medical and enhancement purpose for germline modification? In which category would we put short stature, for example? We know that taller people tend to earn more money. So do people with paler skins. Should arranging for children with financially or socially "efficient" varieties of height and complexion be considered medical intervention? (Darnovsky 2016)

Savulescu proposed the PPB at a time when PGD and IVF were highly debated. New molecular technologies, however, such as CrispR-Cas9, currently permit not only genetic screening but also genetic editing, which actually means making changes to genes. Savulescu envisaged this possibility, saying that, in this case also, parents have the obligation to enhance their children genetically (Savulescu 2001). Overall also contributed a chapter to the book Human Enhancement in 2009 (Overall 2009). Like all her fellow contributors to this volume, she did not mention women's role in this scenario.

In 2008, I noted the glaring absence in a special session on enhancing in the 2006 International Association of Bioethics congress in Beijing (Simonstein 2008b). Overall also became aware of this, and later observed that in Savulescu's discussions of the PPB, he "shockingly" does not refer to women (Overall 2012, p. 125). Overall observes that the PPB proposed by Savulescu refers almost exclusively to "couples" and occasionally to "single reproducers." Nonetheless, she remarks, women are the means of securing the birth of future generations. Women also confront the physical and moral responsibility on reproductive matters. Overall:

> Unlike men…it is the woman who undergoes the physical consequences of conception and pregnancy. Even if she has an abortion…she must bear the moral, pragmatic, and medical weight of making that decision. If she continues the pregnancy, she must care for herself as her body changes radically and must take into account all the consequences of her actions for the fetus. During labor and delivery, she undergoes an experience that can be uniquely demanding and often severely painful. (Overall 2012, p. 9)

All this happens before any genetic manipulation. If the PPB were adopted, it would weigh far more heavily on women than on men because genetic procreative beneficence demands the use of preimplantation diagnosis after in vitro fertilization. This means that every potential mother would be required to undergo this process, and half of the population—the women only—would have to be actively engaged "in a dangerous project" (Overall 2012, p. 126).[5]

Reproductive Risk

As mentioned in previous chapters, reproductive risks have always been part of a woman's life. These risks have diminished in developed countries due to better knowledge and medical care. Would it be fair to add the pain and risks involved in IVF to women's challenging reproductive tasks? As noted in Chap. 7, IVF requires the use of drugs to stimulate the production of multiple ova, following which eggs are removed from the woman's body, fertilized in a Petri dish in the lab, and inserted back into her uterus. Moreover, complications due to IVF have remained underreported. Allegedly, the reason for underreporting is that complications are regarded as part of a "normal" pregnancy; i.e., not necessarily as a result of IVF (see also Chap. 8).

There is no doubt that IVF has become a "routine" procedure through which millions of children worldwide have been born. However, we should bear in mind that these children represent a tiny proportion of success in the general outcome of IVF. Although according to Matti Häyry, the IVF procedure is now "safer" and "more efficient" than it was 30 years ago (Häyry 2010, p. 158), according to other reports, the efficiency of IVF has remained constant. For example, as I noted also

---

[5] PGD is actually necessary to pick the "best" embryos, but occurs among a minority of women, who are undergoing IVF in any case, to overcome fertility. Mostly. There are already cases of women who are doing IVF, not because of infertility, but in order to choose to implant embryos that do not contain the BRC1 and BRC2 genes that cause familial breast cancer.

in the previous chapter, the average success of each round of IVF in Israel, where all women are entitled to IVF free of charge for as long as they are able to bear it, has remained at approximately 16–17% since the mid-1980s (Simonstein et al. 2014). With a probability of more than 80% of failure in each round, IVF has, in fact, become an "experimental" routine. Indeed, as I explored in the previous chapter and noted more than a decade ago IVF is the largest experiment on human subjects in human history (Simonstein 2006).

After 40 years, things have changed for the better, with better drugs, possibly, and better protocols including perhaps in the future "easy PGD" (see above). However, the fact remains that each woman who has a failed attempt with IVF—which, as noted above, happens in around 80% of IVF cycles—becomes a new experiment. In an enhancing scenario, women would be engaging further in a massive medical experiment that includes bodily invasion, time, low success rate, and the risks related to a pregnancy with IVF (Overall 2012).

9.5   Would Women Be Under Pressure to Reproduce with IVF?

The role of women in enhancing reproduction has not yet been discussed by its proponents. However, we may borrow arguments from other enhancing-related discussions to consider how women might fare in an enhancement scenario. Harris, for example, arguing in favor of collaboration in research involving human subjects (not necessarily of women) writes that "danger does not remove our duty to help others." He proposes that when the risks to research subjects "are significant and the burdens onerous but…the benefits to other people are equally significant and large," it would probably be wrong to "force" people to participate; but this "is not to say that individuals should not be willing to bear such burdens nor is it to say that it is not their moral duty to do so". (Harris 2005). The implication of this is that women might have a moral duty to "bear" the burdens of enhancing future generations. Furthermore, if, according to Harris, the inheritance of future generations should be our concern and responsibility, should it become women's responsibility in the case of genetic enhancing? Harris writes that disabling genetic disorders, which could have been prevented, but were not, are "negatively inflicted harms" and, therefore, "immoral." It follows from this view that if a woman opts to reject reproduction with IVF, she would be guilty of wrongdoing. Referring to the lack of consent (by a child who is not yet alive), Harris writes that "allowing genetic harms in future generations due to lack of consent… would [also] be immoral". (Harris 2007, p. 80). Thus, it follows that lack of the mother's consent to reproduce with IVF would be equally morally wrong.

Arguments may be borrowed from additional discussions on enhancing. For instance, in defense of gene-editing research, Savulescu et al. write that it "is not an option, but a moral necessity". (Savulescu et al. 2015, p. 479). Thus, the declaration that gene-editing research is a moral necessity implies that, if it is successful, women, too, might be asked to act "morally." In other words, reproducing with IVF for the sake of enhancing future generations might not merely be an option, but a moral requirement. Savulescu and Kahane might answer that the PPB does not represent the view that reproducers "should be coerced into selecting the most advantaged child, or punished if they don't" (Savulescu and Kahane 2009, p. 279). In their view, the PPB does not allow a government or social agencies to police pregnant women's behavior or make IVF and PGD compulsory. As Solinger rightly observes, however, private decisions about reproduction are always shaped by public laws and policies (Solinger 2005). Solinger points out that this might be a particularly difficult insight to bring into focus, partly because of the way "personal choice" has eclipsed all other ways of thinking about pregnancy and motherhood. In addition, according to Overall, implementing the PPB on a wide scale would affect public policy because "a widely adopted moral principle" regarding human reproduction "cannot be neutral with respect to social action". (Overall 2012, p. 130). Neither can it be assumed that it will not have effects on women's well-being and freedom. Now, in a scenario of genetic enhancing and the PPB, would ensuring women's autonomy and choice require the advent of an artificial womb?

Women's Well-Being and Freedom

When discussing "women's well-being" and "freedom" in reproductive matters, it is impossible to overlook Shulamith Firestone's work during the 1970s (see also Chap. 10). Firestone wrote that technology, i.e., artificial wombs, can liberate women from their biology and extend their choices (Firestone 2003 [1970]). However, according to Pilcher and Whelehan (2005), other feminists claimed that the technological "invasion" of women's bodies by science amounts to a patriarchal strategy to deny women their one advantage over men. This claim has been regarded as overstated, by other feminists who have argued that such interpretation places too much emphasis on "patriarchal" medicine and science while minimizing the knowledge and agency of women themselves (Steinberg 1997). Feminists have also suggested the notion of "relational autonomy;" an idea that takes into account the social "embeddedness" of women's reproductive choices (Sherwin 1998; MacKenzie and Stoljar 2000).

While feminists remain divided on the matter, according to Rosalie Ber (2009), the advent of the artificial womb is not a question of whether it might become available, but a question of when (see also Chap. 10). Moreover, in a scenario of genetic enhancement and the PPB, would ensuring women's autonomy and choice invite the advent of an artificial womb? Tuija Takala, following Firestone, has argued, more recently, that the reason for the ongoing lack of equality between the sexes boils down to the fact that women (and only women) are expected to bear and rear children. Takala claims that women, collectively and individually, should welcome the possibility of nurturing the embryo and fetus outside the womb—ectogenesis—for the length of the entire gestation period (Takala 2009). Firestone's claims in the 1970s, and Takala's 40 years later, were laid regardless of reprogenetics and before Savulescu's suggestion of the PPB. Women's arduous involvement in reproduction was enough to make these claims of these women in favor of artificial wombs. Now, if genetic enhancing were to become safe and the PPB was adopted by society, it would be a gendered project. In such a scenario, women's involvement in reproduction would become even more demanding. Women's well-being and freedom will further diminish unless the artificial womb is developed (see Chaps. 10 and 11).

This chapter is not an exhaustive analysis of the complex issues involved in genetic enhancement. Nonetheless, it offers a clearer picture of a rather elusive future, in which women might be asked to reproduce via IVF for the "betterment" of future generations, a requirement that may herald the advent of the artificial womb. This picture does not necessarily present a slippery slope, but shows the evolving pattern of a long human process of self-awareness and awareness of the world in which we live.[6] There is no doubt about the urgent need for further discussion of the merits and risks of human genome modification, involving scientists, clinicians, social scientists, and the wider public (Baltimore et al. 2015). However, these discussions should include both men *and* women, and clearly spell out the role of women in this scenario.

9.6 Conclusions

This chapter has joined the dots of a rather elusive picture: from a growing mature and aging population in chronic ill health and health care allocation to genetic editing of the germline as a possible solution; from the necessary role of women in a scenario of enhancing future generations to the advent of the artificial womb. Although they do not appear so, these issues are, in fact, connected. Editing the germline to improve the health of future generations might coincide with public health goals; it might improve the health of individuals and communities, and, if successful, might be seen as being for the public good. However, enhancing future generations will require PGD and IVF.

In the context of womb politics, this begs the question of whether all women might have to conceive with IVF. Remarkably, the necessary involvement of women in an enhancing scenario has not been discussed by its proponents. Despite the lack of a unified feminist conclusion in the discussions about the merits and risks of human genome modification, there is an urgent need to clarify the role of women in this scenario. The present discourse on moral obligations to future generations, although not referring to women, seems to imply that women might be required, morally, if not legally, to reproduce with IVF. Since enhancing evolution with gene editing of the germline would be a gendered project—unless the artificial womb is developed—questions about women's role in this scenario must be addressed.

Moreover, the idea of and the reasons for enhancing evolution might *invite* the advent of the artificial womb (AW). The AW and ectogenesis is the focus of the next chapter.

---

[6] For a brilliant account of the evolution of the human race during the last millennia, see: Mortimer, Ian (2014) Human Race: 10 Centuries of Change on Earth. London: Penguin.

Notes

(1) Cyranoski, D. The CRISPR-baby scandal: what's next for human gene-editing. https://www.nature.com/articles/d41586-019-00673-1. Accessed 4 Nov 2020.
(2) Ledford, H. CRISPR gene editing in human embryos wreaks chromosomal mayhem. https://www.nature.com/articles/d41586-020-01906-4. Accessed 3 Nov 2020.
(3) Kennedy, M. Chinese Researcher Who Created Gene-Edited Babies Sentenced to 3 Years in Prison. https://www.npr.org/2019/12/30/792340177/chinese-researcher-who-created-gene-edited-babies-sentenced-to-3-years-in-prison. Accessed 22 Nov 2020.

References

Baltimore, D., M. Berg, M. Botcha, et al. 2015. A Prudent Path Forward for Genomic Engineering and Germline Gene Modification. *Science* 348: 36–38.
Ber, R. 2009. Ethical Issues in Gestational Surrogacy. *Theoretical Medicine and Bioethics* 21: 153–169.
Bostrom, N., and J. Savulescu. 2013 [2009]. Human Enhancement Ethics: The State of the Debate. In *Human Enhancement*, ed. Julian Savulescu and Nick Bostrom, 1–24. Oxford: Oxford University Press.
Darnovsky, M. 2016. Con: Do Not Open the Door to Editing Genes in Future Humans. In *Pro and Con: Should Gene Editing Be Performed on Human Embryos?* National Geographic. https://www.nationalgeographic.com/magazine/2016/08/human-gene-editing-pro-con-opinions/. Accessed 22 Nov 2020.
Firestone, S. 2003 [1970]. *The Dialectic of Sex*. New York: Farrar, Straus and Giroux.
Greely, H.T. 2016. *The End of Sex and the Future of Human Reproduction*. USA: Harvard University Press.
Harris, J. 1993. *Wonderwoman and Superman: The Ethics of Human Biotechnology*. Oxford: Oxford University Press.
Harris, J. 2005. Scientific Research Is a Moral Duty. *Journal of Medical Ethics* 31: 242–248.
Harris, J. 2007. *Enhancing Evolution: The Ethical Case for Making Better People*. Princeton, NJ: Princeton University Press.
Harris, J. 2013 [2009]. Enhancements Are a Moral Obligation. In *Human Enhancement*, ed. Julian Savulescu and Nick Bostrom, 131–154. Oxford: Oxford University Press.
Häyry, M. 2010. *Rationality and the Genetic Challenge: Making People Better?* Cambridge: Cambridge University Press.
MacKenzie, C., and N. Stoljar. 2000. Introduction: Autonomy Refigured. In *Relational Autonomy: Feminist Perspectives on Autonomy, Agency, and the Social Self*, ed. C. MacKenzie and N. Stoljar. Oxford: Oxford University Press.
Overall, C. 2009. Life Enhancement Technologies: Significance of Social Category Membership. In *Human Enhancement*, ed. Julian Savulescu and Nick Bostrom, 327–340. Oxford: Oxford University Press.
Overall, C. 2012. *Why Have Children? The Ethical Debate*. Cambridge, MA: MIT Press.
Pilcher, J., and I. Whelehan. 2005. *50 Key Concepts in Gender Studies*, 3rd ed. London: Sage.
Ran, F.A., P.D. Hsu, J. Wright, et al. 2013. Genome Engineering Using the CRISPR-Cas9 System. *Nature Protocols* 8: 2281–2308.
Savulescu, J. 2001. *"Procreative Beneficence": Why We Should Select the Best Children*. London: Blackwell Publishing.
Savulescu, J. 2006. Genetic Interventions and the Ethics of Enhancement of Human Beings. In *The Oxford Handbook on Bioethics*, ed. Bonnie Steinbock, 516–535. Oxford: Oxford University Press.

Savulescu, J., and G. Kahane. 2009. The Moral Obligation to Create Children with the Best Chance of the Best Life. *Bioethics* 23: 274–290.

Savulescu, J., J. Pugh, T. Douglas, et al. 2015. The Moral Imperative to Continue Gene Editing Research on Human Embryos. *Protein and Cell* 6: 476–479.

Senior, M. 2015. UK Funding Agencies Weigh in on Human Germline Editing. *Nature Biotechnology* 33: 1118–1119.

Sherwin, S. 1998. A Relational Approach to Autonomy in Health Care. In *The Politics of Women's Health: Exploring Agency and Autonomy in Health Care*, ed. Susan Sherwin, 1–28. Philadelphia: Temple University Press.

Silver, M. Lee. 1998. *Remaking Eden*. London: Weidenfeld and Nicolson.

Simonstein, F. 2006. Artificial Reproduction Technologies and Women as Human Subjects for Research. *Medicine and Law* 26: 8–12.

Simonstein, Frida. 2008a. Embryonic Stem Cells: The Disagreement Debate and Embryonic Stem Cell Research in Israel. *Journal of Medical Ethics* 34: 732–734. https://doi.org/10.1136/jme.2007.023549.

Simonstein, F. 2008b. Human Enhancement and Factor X. *Journal of Medical Ethics* 34: 102–103.

Simonstein, F. 2014. *The Ethics of Self-Evolution*. Tel-Aviv: Yozmot.

Simonstein, F., M. Mashiach-Eizenberg, A. Revel, and Y. Yunes. 2014. Assisted Reproduction Policies in Israel: A Retrospective Analysis of IVF-ET. *Fertility and Sterility* 102: 1301–1306.

Solinger, R. 2005. *Pregnancy and Power*. New York: New York University Press.

Steinberg, D. 1997. *Bodies in Glass: Genetics Eugenics and Embryo Ethics*. Manchester: Manchester University Press.

Takala, T. 2009. Human Before Sex? Ectogenesis as a Way to Equality. In *Reprogen-Ethics and the Future of Gender*, ed. Frida Simonstein, 187–196. London: Springer.

Walker, A. 2009. Commentary: The Emergence and Application of Active Aging in Europe. *Journal of Aging and Social Policy* 21: 75–93.

Wang, S., F. Yi, and J. Qu. 2015. Eliminate Mitochondrial Diseases by Gene Editing in Germ-Line Cells and Embryos. *Protein and Cell* 6: 472–475.

XinhuaNet. 2019. He Jiankui Jailed for Illegal Human Embryo Gene-Editing. http://www.xinhuanet.com/english/2019-12/30/c_138666754.htm. Accessed 22 Nov 2020

Zimmer, Z., and S.A. McDaniel. 2013. Global Ageing in the Twenty-First Century. In *Ageing in the Twenty-First Century: Challenges, Opportunities and Implications*, ed. Z. Zimmer and S. McDaniel, 1–12. New York: Ashgate.

Chapter 10
The Artificial Womb (AW)

Imagine for a moment that it is possible to beget children without placing any kind of burden on women. Imagine a world where the health-related risks associated with pregnancy and childbirth have become obsolete. (Cavaliere 2020, p. 76)

Throughout most of human history women have been defined by their biological role in reproduction, seen first and foremost as gestators, which has led to the reproductive system being subjected to outside interference. The womb was perceived as dangerous and an object which husbands, doctors and the state had a legitimate interest in controlling. (Romanis et al. 2020)

In the previous chapter, I noted that reprogenetics, the combination of genetic intervention with assisted reproduction, has produced the idea that genetic improvement—enhancement—of future generations may be feasible. According to some ethicists, the genetic enhancing of future generations—when and if safely achieved—is an ethical imperative (see Chap. 9). The aim of this book is not to join the debate on genetic intervention of the germline for enhancing future generations. The focus of this chapter is on the role expected of women in an enhancing scenario. For if the idea of "benefiting" future generations with genetic enhancement is accepted, all women will have to reproduce via IVF.

So far, the proponents of genetic enhancement have neither mentioned nor referred to the role of women in such a scenario. For the proponents of genetic enhancement of future generations, women's role in reproduction is apparently taken for granted. Women already shoulder the difficulties and perils of natural pregnancies. Adding to this "naturalness," the burdens and perils of conception with IVF is a harsh—and more dangerous—demand from women. Such a scenario may further require—and even invite—the advent of the artificial womb. The idea of an artificial womb and ectogenesis—a child brought to term outside a biological womb—has appeared in various thought experiments (Singer and Wells 1984; Harris 1998; Becker 2017; Strong 2002). Several movies have also shown some frightening scenarios based

This is a revised version of a paper published in Philosophy of Medicine and Health Care 2006 (9) 359–365.

on this idea. Hence many people's initial reaction of revulsion and/or fear when confronted with the suggestion of ectogenesis; and while some medical sources avoid discussion on this topic,[1] others have chosen to address the advent of the artificial womb as a matter of fact (Ber 2000). Those who believe that full pregnancy outside the human body, full ectogenesis, "appears to be a long way off" target the possibility of partial ectogenesis—the supporting of human fetuses during the end part of a pregnancy—under the label of "ectogestation." (Di Stefano et al. 2019).

In the first part of this chapter, I present the scientific and technological research indicating that the advent of the AW may be closer than we think. The focus is on the health toll that reproduction takes on women, which could be avoided through ectogenesis. The final part of the chapter discusses some new conundrums that ectogenesis may entail. I have adopted the term "ectogestation" when referring to the end of a pregnancy, and "ectogenesis" when referring to full gestation outside of a woman's body from the very beginning. While the AW is the tool and ectogenesis the process, in this chapter, I address these terminologies interchangeably.

10.1   Research on Ectogenesis

Neonatal Care

In April 2017, a published article entitled "An artificial womb successfully grew baby sheep—and humans could be next" stated that lambs spent four weeks in "external wombs" and "seemed to develop normally." (Becker 2017). This choice of title followed a paper published in one of the Nature journals, reporting the development of a system that "closely" reproduced the environment of the womb (Partridge et al. 2017). The report explained that "fetal lambs that are developmentally equivalent to the extreme premature human infant can be physiologically supported in an extra-uterine device for up to 4 weeks". (Becker 2017). According to an interview for The Guardian newspaper in the UK, the team who made these artificial wombs claimed that "[they] are driven only by the desire to save the most vulnerable humans on Earth." (Kleeman 2020).

The attempt to save premature neonates is not new. The first special unit for premature infants was opened in 1922; but in 1988 in the United States, 600 hospitals were already providing 7500 NICU beds (Jennings 1988). In 1975, Faye Bland was the first reported baby to survive after being born six months prematurely and weighing only 470 g. At the time, the survival of this baby was considered a medical "accident" since he was not supposed to survive. By the early seventies, doctors focused their efforts on trying to save babies who weighed around 1500 g; and those weighing less than 1000 g were allowed to die because nothing much could be done for them. Moreover, 10 years earlier, nobody would have tried to put a baby as

---

[1] For example, Julian Savulescu at the International Congress on the Ethics of IVF in London during September 2004 asked the scientific panel to refer to ectogenesis. The panelists just ignored the question.

premature as Faye Bland in neonatal care. As Singer and Wells remarkably predicted more than three decades ago, today there is nothing extraordinary about the survival of a newborn weighing 470 g (Singer and Wells 1984).

By 2004, the first databases were tracking outcomes for babies weighing 401–500 g. This weight group of micro preemies was considered "experimental" since mortality in this group approaches 90% (Sills 2003). In that year, the outcome of a 4-year-old girl, Or Iluz, was recorded. She was the tiniest baby who had survived following a birth weight of 300 g, in Israel in 2000 (Eben 2004). In addition, at the beginning of the twenty-first century, the University of Iowa Children's Hospital opened a website registering the world's smallest surviving babies.[1] The infants listed on this website include reports from the lay media and medical journals as well as those submitted directly to the registry by a family member, verified by a health provider. By the end of 2020, the number of premature babies listed, who were born in or before the 24th week of gestation, was 274.[2]

According to this registry, the tiniest infant was born in Tokyo, at 22 weeks, weighing just 246 g; 23 babies were born at 22 weeks, and three were born at 21 weeks. By the end of 2020, Kawagoe in Japan and Cologne in Germany had the highest number of reports on this list. Although reports of babies born at 21 and 22 weeks were made mostly in the last two years, this list included a report of a premature baby born at 21 weeks, dating back to 2006.[1] At the time of writing this chapter, the aforementioned Or Iluz from Israel was not included in this report. It is, therefore, obvious, that more extremely premature babies are being born and kept alive than the 274 listed on the University of Iowa Children's Hospital website. What this listing clearly suggests, however, is that the age of gestation at birth continues to decrease worldwide. Moreover, this registry demonstrates that, globally, there is a huge effort to keep such premature babies—fetuses, in fact—alive.

Indeed, neonatal care has now expanded from caring for neonates, who need only a few hours or days of special care after delivery, to an ever-expanding frontier of prolonged, aggressive treatment for smaller and smaller infants. The trouble is, these infants are dependent on external life support as they move from their mothers' natural wombs to "technological wombs" in a Neonatal Intensive Care Unit (NICU). In Denmark, a consensus has been reached against treating these babies. Yet, in many parts of the world, saving the lives of these babies might be considered an obligatory act.

Savior acts to keep premature babies alive are highly influenced by pro-life campaigners. In addition, some neonatologists observe that they cannot know a priori which of these babies may survive and even get to college (personal communication). Nonetheless, the outcomes of these savior acts are not always encouraging because the improved survival of early and/or extremely low birth weight (ELBWs) and gestational age infants may be accompanied by increased risks of chronic medical problems and neurodevelopmental disabilities (Jennings 1988). As a result, to improve outcomes, neonatologists have thought that an "artificial placenta" could be used. For example, at the American Re-HealthCare Symposium in 2003, Sills, from the Intensive Care Nursery, University of California, clearly expressed this view:

[i]t would be ideal to continue the in uterus environment, keeping the premature infant in a warm water bath (free of infection) attached to its artificial placenta. Under ideal physio-logic conditions the premature would grow and develop normally, free of injury. (Sills 2003)

Back then, Sills was not talking completely "out of the blue." In 1997, Thomas Schaffer at Temple University had developed an amniotic fluid, helping to mimic the way a fetus breathes in the womb. And Yoshinori Kuwabara, a professor of obstetrics at Juntendo University in Japan, had reported actually creating an artificial womb, using an acrylic tank filled with a fluid at body temperature similar to amniotic fluid.[2] This artificial womb had successfully developed goat fetuses to term. The animal fetuses lay submerged in this "tank womb" attached by the umbilical cord to a machine that acted as a placenta, bringing oxygen and nutrients to the fetuses as well as acting as a dialysis machine, cleaning the fetuses' blood.[2]

Therefore, the 2017 publication in Nature about sheep was far from surprising, as this was no longer a novelty. However, this publication attracted the attention of many writers over the AW and ectogenesis. Kingma and Finn (2020), for example, write that ectogenesis is not just "improved neonatal incubation," but "genuine ecto-gestation;" and that "birth" marks "a substantive physiological transition beyond change of location alone, which makes fetuses and neonates very different from each other, regardless of gestational age or level of linear development." In their view, there is "a clear distinction" between "neonatal incubation" and "ectogesta-tion," with the former supporting "neonatal" physiology (by using "ectogenetive" technology), and the latter preserving "fetal" physiology (by using "ectogestative" technology).[2] However, this remains a wishful thought since there is a clear distinc-tion between "neonatal physiology" of fully developed neonates at birth and those neonates that at birth are, in fact, fetuses. Fetuses retain their "fetal physiology" regardless of location, and therefore are in full need of "ectogestative" technology.

There is still some disagreement about what should be done with ELBWs and prematurely born infants because of the huge costs of NICUs, which continue to rise due to novel improvements. Paradoxically, new developments make it possible to save the lives of more ELWBs and more premature babies.[3] This way of pushing back the barriers of neonatal survival is unlikely to end, since sporadic successes have made neonatologists ask questions such as "how small is too small" and "how much is too much" to provide care for preemies at the threshold of viability (Ly 2003; Lee

---

[2] They also suggest not using the term "artificial womb." Kingma, E., Finn, S. (2020). Neonatal incubator or artificial womb? Distinguishing ectogestation and ectogenesis using the metaphysics of pregnancy. Bioethics, 34(4):354–363 (p. 354). But does the name of the technology really matter? There is also a lively discussion on the terminology that should be used for newborns in need of AW technology compared to full-term newborns. See Colgrove, N. (2019). Are subjects of ectogenesis "gestatelings" fetuses, newborns, or neither? Journal of Medical Ethics. 45:723–726; Kingma, E. (2021). In defense of gestatelings: response to Colgrove. Journal of Medical Ethics. 47: 355–356.

[3] Paradoxically, the remarkable success of ARTs is one of the main contributors to NICUs: in Israel, for instance, almost half of the very low birth weight (VLBW) infants admitted to NICUs are the product of ART, and more than a third of VLBW live-born infants are multiple births. VLBW (birth weight less than 1500 g) rates increased from 1.1 to 1.3% of total live births from 1995 to 1998. Between 1993 and 1998, the total number of VLBW infants born each year increased by 40%. See: Zmora E. (2001). Ethics and Neonatology in Israel. *The Journal of Clinical Ethics* 12: 304–307.

et al. 2000; Lorenz 2001; Piecuh et al. 1997). This approach remains controversial because of the morbidity, the suffering, and the huge costs.

The newer databases documenting babies born at less than 300 g clearly demonstrate continuation of this trend. Furthermore, if neonatal morbidity could be avoided, outcries against the huge costs of NICUs would probably disappear. Moreover, some societies are conditioned toward the approval of efforts to save the life of a newborn, no matter its state of health and regardless of the outcomes. Hence the general, generous support for neonatal care. For example, since 2013, Israel has added millions of shekels to neonatal NICU budgets. Most telling is the monetary incentive of twice the yearly monetary support offered to the best five neonatal NICUs in the country.[3] In the guidelines, the word "best" is not clearly defined; evidently though, the survival of newborns—unrelated to weight and prematurity—is a key parameter. As a result, there is a tacit "war" between neonatal NICUs in Israel for neonates' survival. Consequently (and not only in Israel), research in this earliest frontier between life and death has become integral to neonatal care. And since an artificial womb—or "placenta"—may improve outcomes for ELWBs, it remains quite improbable that there could be any obstacle to further development of "ectogestation."

IVF Research

Nevertheless, research at the beginning of gestation is viewed very differently. While research activity on embryos at the end of gestation is supported generously because it may save the lives of tiny humans, research at the beginning of gestation has been controversial. Indeed, research at this stage of development has been highly contentious. In most countries, research on embryos beyond day 14 after fertilization is banned. For example, in 1993, Canada explicitly prohibited "any experimentation which may lead to ectogenesis." (Proceed with Care Final Report of the Royal Commission on New Reproductive Technologies 1993). Yet the report for artificial reproduction regulations equally exhorted for better results in IVF cycles. This cannot be pursued without further research on the process of embryo implantation in the womb which, obviously, is experimentation that may lead to ectogenesis.

It follows that the 1993 proposal for ARTs regulations in Canada was incoherent. Moreover, improving rates of IVF in the United States has also become a competitive target in a free market, so IVF fertility clinics are under pressure to publish their success rates. And rightly so, since this demand may improve IVF effectiveness, reduce both the costs of IVF and women's suffering (see Chap. 7).[4] Three decades ago, Professor Hung-Ching Liu from Cornell University explained the need for this research:

> Human in vitro fertilization is characterized by a low efficiency of implantation …Embryo viability or quality, abnormal implantation and delayed or absent corpus luteum rescue may all play a role in pregnancy wastage. Defining the possible mechanism for these losses may allow hormonal treatment to correct specific abnormalities. (Liu and Rosenwaks 1991)

Therefore, Liu and her team grew a human uterus by taking endometrial cells over scaffolding in the shape of a uterus. The scaffolding dissolved as the cells grew into

---

[4] The rate of implantation is low in nature as well. Yet the natural process is cheaper and painless.

uterine tissue, and the womb was then supplied with proper nutrients and hormones. To test the womb, embryos left over from IVF programs were introduced, and actually began to settle properly. The experiment was halted after six days.

Obviously, improvements in IVF cannot be made without research on embryo implantation in the uterus. Yet since the implant of embryo research must mimic the process in the womb, there can be little doubt that this is research on ectogenesis. Liu, then, was not shy on this matter. During the congress of the American Society of Reproductive Medicine, in Orlando, Florida in 2001, she claimed that her final goal was "having a child in the laboratory." In the coverage of the 2004 OBYGIN conference she explained as follows:

> … I want to see whether I can develop an actual external device and then with a computer system simulate the feed in medium, feed out medium…and have a chip controlling the hormonal level…I believe if this can be achieved, we could possibly have an artificial uterus so then you could grow a baby to term.[4] (Liu cited in Alghran 2018, p. 122)

Neonatologists—and many others—addressed Liu's "vision" as the views of a deranged scientist, a lonely "cowboy." (Alghran 2018). Notwithstanding Liu's good reputation in her field as Director of the Reproductive Endocrine Laboratory at the Center for Reproductive Medicine and Infertility at Cornell University and as one of the world's leading researchers in reproductive endocrinology. By 2004, she had published more than 70 peer-reviewed articles in medical publications and had delivered more than a hundred presentations on research topics at medical meetings around the world.[5] However, since that conference, Liu refused to answer questions on the matter (personal communication). At the time of writing this chapter, the website that addressed Liu's words in 2004 remains at Cornell University, but the specific page no longer exists. Nevertheless, her profile can be found in academic networks such as Research Gate (with 171 publications)[6] and LinkedIn.[7]

Professor Hung-Ching Liu may have retired. With her departure, research at the first stages of embryo implant in the womb—ectogenesis—might have disappeared. Nonetheless, on June 12, 2019, on the first page of the weekend supplement of an Israeli newspaper, a somewhat awkward title appeared: "Professor, Make Me a Child". (Rozenblum 2019). This article told the story of an ongoing research about an artificial womb, pursued by Professor Dan Grisaru from Ichilov Hospital in Israel. According to this reportage, Grisaru and his team had claimed being close to a breakthrough "that could change the world." (Rozenblum 2019). They were planning to print an entire womb outside the body, which could allow babies to grow in the lab until their artificial birth. The female science reporter, Rosenblum, writes, with apparent excitement:

> Imagine [having] a baby without pregnancy and childbirth; without the doubt of whether there is a pregnancy or not, without the painful tests, without the severe pain of childbirth. This could be the humankind fertility world a few years ahead. (Rozenblum 2019, p. 34)

Rosenblum may be wrong. However, Grisaru is the Director of the Oncology and Gynecology Unit at Ichilov Hospital in Tel Aviv and a faculty member at Tel Aviv University. Together with Professor David Elhad from the Bioengineering Faculty of

Tel Aviv University and their team, they had already published a paper in a journal of the Nature Group, reporting successful growth of womb tissue in the lab (Kuperman et al. 2020). Thus, even if Professor Liu from Columbia University has retired, her line of research survives.

Embriology Research

Neonatologists, at this point, would rightly observe that the gap between week 22 and the second gestational week is insuperable. The lungs of very premature babies collapse, their blood vessels bleed easily, causing damage, particularly in the brain, and infections and death are common. However, barriers that seem insuperable today are only temporary obstacles. Indeed, embryo development has been at the center of arduous research since the second half of the twentieth century. Since then, one of the most intriguing questions in biology has been how a cell in a pre-embryo "knows" what to become, when, and where. Most of these questions have remained unanswered; yet this is a puzzle that embryologists are determined to resolve.

For example, Duane Alexander (who, at the beginning of the twenty-first century, was Director of the National Institute of Child Health and Human Development in the United States), claimed in the Foreword for the Strategic Plan 2000, entitled From Cells to Selves, that the task of the Institute for the next years was "to fully understand human embryology." In his words:

> To us falls the task not of curing a single disease or group of diseases but of solving the fundamental question in biology and all that derives from it: how does a single fertilized egg develop into a fully functional adult human being, and how do a multitude of genetic and environmental factors influence that process for good or for ill. Thus the title of this plan: "From Cells to Selves." (Alexander 2000)

Among other areas for "Immediate Strategic Review" in this plan of research for the new millennium was "Developmental Biology," which "should understand Normal and Abnormal Development:" This topic included "the basic biological science necessary to understand early development in utero, and through the time when many organ systems form." (Alexander 2000).

Although research on human embryos after 14 days has been banned in most countries, research on animal embryos has not. Research on animal embryos has already shown that hormones and/or their proportion in solution may develop one organ rather than the other. Frog embryos, for instance, may generate a second head when a specific hormone is more concentrated in the solution; alternatively, a different set of hormones may regenerate other parts of the body. In turn, findings that may arise from stem cell research promote further advancement on the knowledge leading to embryo development (Wilmut and Dominsky 2000; Ahn et al. 2004; Brandenberger et al. 2004).[5] In stem cell research, this knowledge has permitted cell differentiation into different types of tissue. The Human Genome Project, after mapping the human genome, started the process of decoding what a gene does, when, and what for. As the Strategic Plan 2000, "From Cells to Selves," explained:

---

[5] This list is not exhaustive.

> Once the human genome is mapped, the advances will be expansive. Even within a couple of years, the mapping will provide scientists with the "bricks and mortar" they need to understand the intricate programs for turning genes on and off – just at the right moment, in the right sequence, and triggering "back-up circuitry." (Alexander 2000)

This is the idea that has been used to grow tissue in the lab for organ transplants. Kidneys, heart tissue, and hairy skin have already been grown from pluripotent cells (Goto et al. 2019; Lemme et al. 2018; Lee et al. 2018). However, these are also the questions relevant to understanding embryo development and ectogenesis.

Computer science has also been fully adopted by molecular biology research in order to understand protein structure and function. Thus, full ectogenesis, from its very beginning, may become a reality in mammals sooner than we think. Indeed, in some medical circles, the advent of the artificial womb is just a matter of time. For example, Rosalie Ber, MD, Emeritus Professor and ex-Director of Education at the Technion Medical School in Israel, wrote the following two decades ago:

> In view of the de-personalization of the gestational surrogate mother who functions as a "womb for rent" why not permit using the wombs of women in persistent vegetative state [PVS], female bodies kept viable by artificial means, *until technological perfection of an artificial womb is achieved*? (Ber 2000) (my italics).

I will not address Ber's suggestion on PVS here. My focus is that Ber appeared to be certain that the technological perfection of an artificial womb will be achieved, eventually. While Ber's premise was that the technological perfection of an artificial womb was in its "elementary stages" (Ber 2000), the latest development on both sides of gestation, at its end (ectogestation) and at its beginning (ectogenesis), demonstrates that research on AWs—against a worldwide chorus of disapproval—has continued, and serious improvements have been made.

10.2   Reproductive Hazards

So far, the incentive for developing the AW is to save the lives of very premature babies, to improve embryo implant in IVF, and to grow tissues and organs for transplant. Remarkably, absent from the aims of the AW research is the improvement of women's health. The so-called "reproductive hazards" have traditionally been viewed as women's fate and taken for granted. Taking this view, Cook, Dickens, and Fathalla explain candidly that "maternity is not a disease," but "an essential function that women fulfill for the survival of our species." (Cook et al. 2003, p. 29). The problem with this definition of maternity is that although it is not a disease, it is not exactly healthy, and IVF is even riskier. According to the WHO, in 2017, about 300,000 women died during and following pregnancy and childbirth.[8] In that year, 822 women per day died because of a pregnancy. This means that a woman dies in or soon after childbirth every two minutes (!); and although most deaths due to reproductive labor occur in developing countries, according to the CDC, about

700 women die each year in the *United States* as a result of pregnancy or delivery complications.[9]

The argument against these shocking statistics of women still dying in the twenty-first century because of "reproductive hazards" is that most of these deaths, with suitable health provision, may be preventable. However, even without a death sentence (as it has been so many times through human history), for too many women, pregnancy itself still entails bad health. For example, the website of the Centers for Disease Control (CDC) in the United States explains that "Pregnancy symptoms and complications of pregnancy… are *health problems* that occur during pregnancy" (my italics).[10] These "problems" can range from "mild and annoying discomforts" to "severe, sometimes life-threatening, illnesses."[9] The list of pregnancy symptoms and complications at the CDC includes urinary tract infections, mental health conditions, hypertension, gestational diabetes, obesity and weight gain, infections, hyperemesis gravidarum (persistent nausea and vomiting several times during the day), preeclampsia (hypertension also affecting other vital organs), and more, and 20% of all pregnancies end in natural abortion.[10] Furthermore, under the title of "Body Changes and Discomforts" in a pregnancy (meaning "non-health" issues), the CDC explains:

> Everyone expects pregnancy to bring an expanding waistline. But many women are surprised by the other body changes that pop up. Get the low-down on stretch marks, weight gain, heartburn and other "joys" of pregnancy. (Quotation marks in the source).[10]

The list of "discomforts" at the CDC include body aches, breast changes, constipation, dizziness, fatigue, sleep problems, hemorrhoids, itching, leg cramps, morning sickness, nasal problems, numb or tingling hands, skin changes, swelling, urinary frequency and leaking, and varicose veins.[10] Each of these so-called "discomforts" would be considered a health concern, requiring a visit to the GP, in a non-pregnant individual. In the case of a pregnant woman, however, these issues are negligible, normal, merely a pregnancy-related "discomfort," not meriting further attention. Smajdor (2007) points out that if any disease caused the same problems, we would regard them as very serious.

Following Firestone back in 1970, Smajdor claimed that "pregnancy is barbaric." (Smajdor 2007). In a recent interview for The Guardian, Smajdor said that women's suffering during and after pregnancy (incontinence, for example), is not "adequately recognised," as it is all "tied up" with "the strong value we attach not just to motherhood but to giving birth." (cited in Kleeman 2020). There is an unquestioned assumption that women will have babies and thus, we fail to notice "how bizarre it is that women have to produce new human beings out of their bodies; and how dangerous it is." According to Smajdor, our attitude to birth is very strange: "There is blood, pain and stitching even if all goes well, and we are meant to ignore it." (cited in Kleeman 2020). Indeed, as I have pointed out throughout this book, women are largely preconditioned to have babies, and as quietly and uncomplainingly as possible. We ignore the blood, the pain, and the stitches because that is the way things are. Firestone and

Smajdor are very brave when referring to women's reproductive tolls as "barbaric," since this is something about which women are not supposed to complain.[6]

Many women may disagree with this blunt adjective and might add that they enjoyed their role in a pregnancy. Nevertheless, the interviewer admits, after hearing Smajdor, that she had never before thought to question her reproductive role until she heard the provocative ideas used by Smajdor to raise difficult questions. These ideas made her think about how "messed up" our notions of "normal" childbirth, pregnancy, and motherhood are. Kleeman, wrote as follows:

> Pregnancy is remarkable, but I have never felt more like a thing being acted on by doctors. I have definitely felt like an ectogenetic gestator… I have had to lie back while a 20 cm needle was plunged into my belly so doctors could extract my son's DNA because something on a scan made them think he might have Down's syndrome…I have had to lie with my legs clamped apart while a surgeon stitched up my cervix because a scan showed I was at risk of going into another early labour… Being pregnant is a remarkable experience, and I loved carrying my first child, but I have never felt more like a thing, being acted upon… (Kleeman 2020)

Kleeman is careful to mention the "remarkable" experience of pregnancy many times in her report. This is what "good" women are supposed to feel. Nevertheless, the latest news of a possible advent of an AW, in addition to Smajdor's blunt opinions on what a pregnancy entails, made her rethink her role in reproduction. Her afterthoughts about her pregnancy resonated with my own experience. One does not question our reproductive toll because that is the way things are. And, as Kendal reminds us, the only way to avoid pregnancy discomfort, labor pain, and birth trauma has been abstention from pregnancy and childbirth (Kendal 2015). Women's societal conditioning to have babies—still obligatory in some parts of the world—does the rest.

10.3 Facing Ectogenesis

Ectogenesis, if one day proved to be safe, might first be a solution to avoid the need for a surrogate; for women who want a biological baby but lack a womb (for any reason), and for homosexual male couples. It might also, perhaps, appeal to women, who may need IVF to reproduce; women may save time, pain, bad moods, and endless frustration (when embryos fail to implant, for instance). Most importantly, it may prevent damage to women's health; for, as seen above, a pregnancy is not considered an illness (Cook et al. 2003) but neither is it a healthy condition.

Ectogenesis may also, finally, achieve women's equality. As MacKay asserts, "ectogenesis has the potential to challenge traditional patriarchal family structures, and thence all other male-dominated structures (of work, education, cultural production)."[7] However, this claim is contested. Cavaliere, for example, does not believe

---

[6] The first sin in the Bible, anybody?

[7] MacKay, K. (2020). The 'tyranny of reproduction': Could ectogenesis further women's liberation? Bioethics, 34 (4) 346–353.

that ectogenesis could change the present status quo (Cavaliere 2020). In addition, Horn and Romanis (2020) regard MacKay's assumption as "problematic" because it locates the problem of inequity in gendered care labor "in the gestating body," rather than "in the institutional structures that produce it." Nevertheless, a woman who wants a child, with the advent of the AW, might not necessarily be forced to slow down her career because of a pregnancy. And although gender inequality results mainly from childcare, and is not necessarily because of the pregnancy, its roots may be found in the fact that women (unlike men) are those who bear the child and therefore must slow down.[8]

Other authors claim that the idea of an AW has the potential to "exacerbate the notion of maternal–fetus conflict," in which the interests of a pregnant woman and her fetus are presented as "incompatible with, or in competition with, each other." (Romanis et al. 2020). This claim tries to defend the role of women as "good" gestators in reproduction. Sadly, this conflict between the fetus and its mother is a biologic fact, since the purely biologic definition of a human fetus is "parasite." As such, the fetus feeds earnestly on its host. By definition, a parasite, when exploiting its host, also causes harm. In the case of an embryo, it must numb the immune system of its mother to implant in her womb. To avoid expulsion—as a foreign body—the fetus continues downplaying its mother's immune system. If successful in the attack against its mother's immune system, the fetus is expelled from her body only nine months later. We call this expulsion "giving birth" or "childbirth." A newcomer has joined the human race.

A new baby is a welcome event in all human societies. No wonder society has romanticized and idealized women's role in pregnancy. Indeed, the non-romantic biologic fact that a pregnancy is a host–parasite structure is rarely mentioned. Nevertheless, authors (Cavaliere 2020) writing that the "maternal–fetus conflict" is just a social construct—against pregnant women—should at least acknowledge the biologic basis of the conflict. More importantly, the *real* social construct of this conflict is the protection of the fetus only—the attacker—completely forgoing the protection of its host; a woman. As noted above, the protection of women's health is not included in the aims of AW research. Nevertheless, even as a bypass of the actual research aims, the advent of the AW may finally help women to avoid the "health hazards" produced by carrying future generations in their bodies for the sake of humanity.

New Conundrums

The effects that the advent of the AW may have on current legislature (when fully developed and deemed safe) are huge. First, ectogestation may erode present abortion rights (Brassington 2009), which are rooted in a woman's right over her body, till

---

[8] Interestingly, the male and female of a certain breed of fish in the Amazon River can equally feed their offspring from a gland that both carry on their heads. Farias IP, Willis S, Leão A, Verba JT, Crossa M, Foresti F, et al. (2019) The largest fish in the world's biggest river: Genetic connectivity and conservation of *Arapaima gigas* in the Amazon and Araguaia-Tocantins drainages. PLoS ONE 14(8): e0220882. https://doi.org/10.1371/journal.pone.0220882.

viability.[11],[12],9 Viability due to enhanced neonatal procedures is expanding, thus limiting the time for a woman to get an abortion. For example, David Steel, the former liberal leader who introduced Britain's modern abortion laws, called in 2004 for a dramatic reduction in the legal limit for most terminations from 24 to 12 weeks. His Abortion Act of 1967 (regarded as one of the most significant social advances in the post-war period), legalized abortions up to 28 weeks of pregnancy. In 1990, amid concerns that a 28-week-old fetus could survive outside the womb, the limit was cut to 24 weeks. And in 2004, Lord Steel reportedly felt that the time had come to go further, "given the advance of technology." (Watt 2004).

Thus, if ectogenesis were to become a new way to have babies, embryos would be viable from the beginning of a pregnancy. If this were the case, according to the present legislation in some countries (where abortion is permitted), women may not be allowed to abort at all. Still, there are differences between different regional frameworks and from country to country. For example, the Supreme Court of Canada established that protection of the unborn cannot be conferred before meeting the cumulative requirements of the "born, alive and viable" rule. This rule entirely precludes both the interests of the unborn and the public interest from intruding into women's private sphere (Dakic 2019).

Nonetheless, under the national statutes in Europe, viability is the threshold for the commencement of abortion constraints. Thus, after reaching the stage of viability, the rights and interests of the unborn are strictly protected, narrowing down the list of legitimizing grounds for their infringement (Dakic 2019). Furthermore, some countries in Europe are more liberal than others. In England, two doctors have to agree that the mother's mental or physical state could be damaged by continuing with the pregnancy.[13] But in Cyprus, Poland, Portugal, Spain, and Switzerland, abortion laws remain very restrictive, allowing abortion only in cases of rape or fetal impairment, or to protect a woman's physical or mental health.[14]

Another problem is that nature reacts to gross genetic errors with natural miscarriages (Marchetti et al. 2004), in which people cannot interfere since they happen "naturally." But pulling the plug because of a possible human error in the proceedings of ectogenesis will be considered "euthanasia," currently outlawed in most countries. From a different angle, the Supreme Court of Canada case law that excludes both the interest of the unborn and the public interest from intruding into a woman's private matter may be interpreted in such a way that neither technologically induced viability nor artificial conflict elimination could affect the scope of reproductive choice. According to this interpretation, prospective parents would be free to demand interruption of the process to avoid parenthood (Dakic 2019).

One of the most troubling questions about ectogenesis is psychological harm to the child. This question was also asked in the context of IVF. For example, in the recommendations section of the 2004 report of the President's Council on Bioethics,

---

9 See also Romanis E.C. (2021). Abortion & 'artificial wombs': would 'artificial womb' technology legally empower non-gestating genetic progenitors to participate in decisions about *how* to terminate pregnancy in England and Wales? Journal of Law and the Biosciences 8(1):1–36; Romanis, E.C. (2020). Sally Sheldon and Kaye Wellings (eds), Decriminalising Abortion in the UK: What Would It Mean? Medical Law Review.

the council recommends a federally funded longitudinal study of the impact of ARTs on the health and development of children born with their aid (A Report of the President's Council on Bioethics 2004). So far, IVF children seem to be as normal as other children and remain unconcerned about the method by which they were conceived. Similarly, a child born prematurely, who spent months in an incubator, is not considered "different" because society accepts this method of keeping a fetus alive. It is not implausible to think, therefore, that if society accepts ectogenesis, the ectogenetic child could be considered as any other child.

Finally, ectogenesis will be costly; high-tech and round-the-clock care might be a very expensive commodity, affordable only to women (and men) of financial means. One of the claims in favor of ectogenesis is equality and freedom for women. However, some authors contend that ectogenesis is likely to benefit "a small subset of women" and not the group "who most need equality and freedom." (Cavaliere 2020). This notwithstanding, surrogacy, which is also expensive, is permitted in most countries.[10] While many surrogacy agreements have moved from the United States to less expensive countries in Asia and Eastern Europe, they remain costly.[11] Interestingly, ethical concerns of surrogacy go beyond the fact that it is affordable only to the rich. In Canada, for example, surrogacy has been prohibited because using women as "a womb for rent" may lead to abuse of poor women. If this is the case, with ectogenesis, the "need" for a woman who is willing to "rent" her womb to people of financial means disappears; together with the abuse factor.

Nevertheless, it is unlikely that ectogenesis will be covered by any health insurance, as has happened with IVF. Unless, perhaps, grounded proof shows it to be completely safe for the fetus and that avoiding reproductive activity would greatly improve women's health. This study has not been worth conducting since there has been no alternative way to have children. Indeed, women had babies even when the consequences were frequently fatal, before hygiene, antibiotics, and cesarean sections became available. Until the recent advent of the pill, women did not have the choice of whether or not to become pregnant in the first place. Is such a study necessary, though? After all, as mentioned above, the health hazards during and following a pregnancy are bad enough.

---

[10] For example, a British homosexual couple hired a surrogate mother in the US to deliver them twin babies. They were millionaires and so they could afford it. The case became public because by the existing legislature, the babies could not enter the UK. The couple had then to request the intervention of the interior minister.

[11] This is "a new-old" way of reproduction. For example, biblical Sarah used her maid Hagar as a surrogate to have a baby from Abraham. Even in the twentieth century, in countries where the number of children per woman remained high, it was commonplace for a woman who had many children to give her own new baby to a barren sister (personal communication).

10.4   Conclusions

The AW has been the focus of arduous research and might become a reality sooner than we think, as developments in neonatal care, gynecology, embryology, computer science, and the human genome project are converging to this end. The latest developments show that improvements have been made both at the beginning and the end of gestation. Although a huge gap remains in between, the history of science tell us that impenetrable barriers are only temporary. It is only a matter of time (and research) until someone—either intentionally or by chance—finds a way to overcome an obstacle. Despite the apparent existence of too many barriers in the case of the artificial womb, it would be naïve to suppose that things may develop differently than in past scientific breakthroughs.

In the context of womb politics, the challenges that ectogenesis may entail regarding present ethics and legislation may be huge. A wider discussion on this topic seems to have started, when we still have time to decide what we may want and why. Presently, the aims of research toward the AW are to improve neonatal care for very premature babies, to achieve better embryo implantation in IVF, and to grow tissues and organs in the lab for transplant. Remarkably, not included in AW research is the aim of relieving women of the health hazards and "discomforts" that they currently endure in reproduction. The romantic view of pregnancy and childbirth and the societal conditioning of women to have babies remain fully at work.

Supposing that we achieve full, and safe, ectogenesis, it is quite improbable that this societal conditioning of women toward a gendered biological predetermination, over eons of time, would come to an abrupt end. Many (or most?) women would choose to make a baby in "the old way" at least once. For some women, however, the option to have a genuine choice of whether (or not) to bear a child in order to become a parent could be of value.

The next chapter presents a pilot study of lay people's views on the advent of the artificial womb and ectogenesis.

Notes

(1)   Tiniest Babies Registry. https://webapps1.healthcare.uiowa.edu/TiniestBabies/index.aspx. Accessed 27 Dec 2020.
(2)   http://www.w-cpc.org/news/reuter7-97.html. Accessed 13 July 2004.
(3)   https://www.health.gov.il/hozer/mr52_2013.pdf. Accessed 15 Feb 2021.
(4)   OBGYN.net Conference Coverage. http://www.obgyn.net/. Accessed 13 July 2004.
(5)   http://www.ivf.org/liu.html. Accessed 13 July 2004.
(6)   https://www.researchgate.net/profile/Hung-Ching_Liu. Accessed 18 Jan 2021.
(7)   https://www.linkedin.com/in/hung-ching-liu-33b546a1/. Accessed 18 Jan 2021.
(8)   https://www.who.int/news-room/fact-sheets/detail/maternal-mortality. Accessed 8 Mar 2021.
(9)   https://www.cdc.gov/reproductivehealth/maternalinfanthealth/pregnancy-relatedmortality. htm. Accessed 8 Mar 2021.

(10)   https://www.womenshealth.gov/pregnancy/youre-pregnant-now-what/body-changes-and-discomforts. Accessed 8 Mar 2021.
(11)   http://www.canadianlawsite.com/abortion-laws.htm. Accessed 2 Apr 2019.
(12)   http://www.ippf.org/regions/europe/choices/v28n2/legislation.htm. Accessed 2 Apr 2019.
(13)   http://www.nhsdirect.nhs.uk/. Accessed 21 Aug 2004.
(14)   https://www.ippfen.org/resource/ippf-en-partner-survey-abortion-legislation-and-its-imp lementation-europe-and-central-asia.   https://www.europarl.europa.eu/thinktank/en/search. html?keywords=004504. Accessed 6 Feb 2021.

References

A Report of the President's Council on Bioethics. 2004. *Reproduction and Responsibility. The Regulation of New Biotechnologies*, 208. Washington, DC. https://bioethicsarchive.georgetown. edu/pcbe/reports/reproductionandresponsibility/index.html. Accessed 6 Feb 2021.

Ahn, J.I., K.H. Lee, D.M. Shin, et al. 2004. Comprehensive Transcriptome Analysis of Differentiation of Embryonic Stem Cells into Midbrain and Hindbrain Neurons. *Developmental Biology* 265: 491–501.

Alexander, D. 2000. *Foreword From Cells to Selves Strategic Plan 2000.* National Institute of Child Health and Human Development. http://www.nichd.nih.gov/strategicplan/cells.

Alghran, A. 2018. *Regulating Assisted Reproductive Technologies: New Horizons.* Cambridge: Cambridge University Press.

Becker, R. 2017. An Artificial Womb Successfully Grew Baby Sheep—And Humans Could Be Next. https://www.theverge.com/2017/4/25/15421734/artificial-womb-fetus-biobag-uterus-lamb-sheep-birth-premie-preterm-infan. Accessed 18 Mar 2021.

Ber, R. 2000. Ethical Issues in Gestational Surrogacy. *Theoretical Medicine and Bioethics* 21: 153–169.

Brandenberger, R., H. Wei, S. Zhang, S. Lei, J. Murage, et al. 2004. Transcriptome Characterization Elucidates Signaling Networks That Control Human ES Cell Growth and Differentiation. *Nature Biotechnology* 22: 707–716.

Brassington, I. 2009. The Glass Womb. In *Reprogen-Ethics and the Future of Gender*, ed. Frida Simonstein. London: Springer.

Cavaliere, G. 2020. Gestation, Equality and Freedom: Ectogenesis as a Political Perspective. *Journal of Medical Ethics* 46: 76–82.

Cook, R., B.M. Dickens, and M.F. Fathalla. 2003. *Reproductive Health and Human Rights.* New York: Oxford University Press.

Dakic, D. 2019. The Scope of Reproductive Choice and Ectogenesis: A Comparison of European Regional Frameworks and Canadian Constitutional Standards. *ELTE Law Journal* 2: 128–143. https://eltelawjournal.hu/wp-content/uploads/2019/02/10_Drakic.pdf.

Di Stefano, L., C. Mills, A. Watkins, and D. Wilkinson. 2019. Ectogestation Ethics: The Implications of Artificially Extending Gestation for Viability, Newborn Resuscitation and Abortion. *Bioethics.* https://doi.org/10.1111/bioe.12682. Accessed 17 Mar 2021.

Eben, D. 2004. Numbers on Premature Babies. *Saturday Supplement Maariv Newspaper*, 16 July: 2 (in Hebrew).

Firestone, S. 2003 [1970]. *The Dialectic of Sex: The Case for Feminist Revolution.* US: Farrar Straus and Giroux.

Goto, Teppei, Hiromasa Hara, Makoto Sanbo, Hideki Masaki, Hideyuki Sato, et al. 2019. Generation of Pluripotent Stem Cell-Derived Mouse Kidneys in Sall1-Targeted Anephric Rats. *Nature Communications* 10 (1). https://doi.org/10.1038/s41467-019-08394-9.

Harris, J. 1998. *Clones, Genes and Immortality.* Oxford: Oxford University Press.

Horn, C., E.C. Romanis. 2020. Establishing Boundaries for Speculation About Artificial Wombs, Ectogenesis, Gender, and the Gestating Body. In: Dietz, C., Travis, M., Thomson, M. (eds) A Jurisprudence of the Body. Palgrave Socio-Legal Studies. Palgrave Macmillan, Cham, p. 227.

Jennings, B. 1988. Beyond the Right of the Newborn. *Raritan* 7: 79–93.

Kendal, Evie. 2015. *Equal Opportunity and the Case for State Sponsored Ectogenesis*. Basingstoke: Palgrave Macmillan.

Kleeman, J. 2020. 'Parents Can Look at Their Foetus in Real Time': Are Artificial Wombs the Future?, 27 Jun 2020. https://www.theguardian.com/lifeandstyle/2020/jun/27/parents-can-look-foetus-real-time-artificial-wombs-future. Accessed 20 Jan 2021.

Kuperman, T., D. Elad, D. Grisaru, et al. 2020. Tissue-Engineered Multi-Cellular Models of the Uterine Wall. *Biomechanics and Modeling in Mechanobiology* 19: 1629–1639.

Lee, S.K., D.D. McMillan, A. Ohlson, et al. 2000. Variations in Practice and Outcomes in the Canadian NICU Network: 1996–1997. *Pediatrics* 106: 1070–1079.

Lee, Jiyoon, Robert Böscke, Pei-Ciao Tang, Byron H. Hartman, Stefan Heller, et al. 2018. Hair Follicle Development in Mouse Pluripotent Stem Cell-Derived Skin Organoids. *Cell Reports* 22 (1): 242.

Lemme, Marta, Bärbel M. Ulmer, Marc D. Lemoine, Antonia T.L. Zech, Frederik Flenner, et al. 2018. Atrial-Like Engineered Heart Tissue: An In Vitro Model of the Human Atrium. *Stem Cell Reports*. https://doi.org/10.1016/j.stemcr.2018.10.008.

Liu, H.C., and Z. Rosenwaks. 1991. Early Pregnancy Wastage in IVF (In Vitro Fertilization) Patients. *Journal of Assisted Reproduction and Genetics* 8: 65–72.

Lorenz, J.M. 2001. The Outcome of Extreme Prematurity. *Seminars in Perinatology* 25: 348–359.

Ly, H. 2003. Perinatal Care at the Threshold of Viability—From Principles to Practice. *Annals of the Academy of Medicine, Singapore* 32: 362–375.

Marchetti, F., J.B. Bishop, L. Cosentino, et al. 2004. Paternally Transmitted Chromosomal Aberrations in Mouse Zygotes Determine Their Embryonic Fate. *Biology of Reproduction* 70: 616–624.

Partridge, E.A., M.G. Davey, M.A. Hornick, and A.W. Flake. 2017. An EXTrauterine Environment for Neonatal Development: EXTENDING Fetal Physiology Beyond the Womb. *Seminars in Fetal and Neonatal Medicine* 22 (6): 404–409.

Piecuh, R.E., C.H. Leonard, B.A. Cooper, and S.A. Sehring. 1997. Outcome of Extremely Low Birth Weight Infants (500–999 Grams) Over a 12-Year Period. *Pediatrics* 100: 633–639.

Proceed with Care Final Report of the Royal Commission on New Reproductive Technologies. 1993. Minister of Government Services, Canada. Ottawa: Canada Communications Group. Recommendation 184: 637.

Romanis, E.C., D. Begović, M.R. Brazier, et al. 2020. Reviewing the Womb. *Journal of Medical Ethics*. Published Online First: 29 July 2020. https://doi.org/10.1136/medethics-2020-106160. https://jme.bmj.com/content/early/2020/07/28/medethics-2020-106160.info. Accessed 10 Jan 2021.

Rozenblum, S. 2019. Making Life. 7 Days Supplement. *Yediyot Aharonot*, Apr 12: 34 (Hebrew).

Sills, J. 2003. Understanding Catastrophic Health Care Exposures. Neonatal Intensive Care—How Did We Get Here and Where Are We Going? In *American Re-HealthCare Symposium 2003*. http://www.amre.com/hc2003/summaries/sills.htm. Accessed 23 Mar 2004.

Singer, P., and D. Wells. 1984. *The Reproduction Revolution. New Ways to Making Babies*. Oxford: Oxford University Press.

Smajdor, A. 2007. The Moral Imperative for Ectogenesis. *Cambridge Quarterly of Healthcare Ethics* 16 (3): 336–345.

Strong, C. 2002. Overview: A Framework for Reproductive Ethics. In *Ethical Issues in Maternal-Fetal Medicine*, ed. Dona L. Dickenson, 17–36. Cambridge: Cambridge University Press.

Watt, N. 2004. Steel Calls for Abortion Limit to Be Cut. *The Guardian*, 5 July. http://society.guardian.co.uk/. Accessed online 5 July 2004.

Wilmut, I., and T. Dominsky. 2000. Editorial. Government Encouragement for Therapeutic Cloning. *Cloning* 2: 53–54.

Chapter 11
A Survey of Lay People's Attitudes Toward the Artificial Womb and Ectogenesis in Israel

As I suggested in the previous chapter, the artificial womb (AW) and ectogenesis—a child brought to term outside a biological womb—may become a reality sooner than we think. As I noted in Chap. 10 and elsewhere (Simonstein 2006), research in disparate areas (such as neonatal care, assisted reproduction, embryology, fetal surgery, computer science and the human genome project) is converging to this end. Society is also pushing in this direction. Society, at large, aims to save very premature newborns and demands better outcomes in IVF. Because of this pressure, both ends of the gestation process, its commencement (conception) and culmination (very premature birth), are undergoing a massive research effort. While a huge gap remains between the first stages of gestation (by IVF) and the 22nd week of gestation (inside the womb), it is plausible that this gap will eventually be overcome. Recent advances in ectogestation for very premature babies (Partridge et al. 2017) and successful developments of AWs from scratch (Kuperman et al. 2020) prove that ectogenesis is on the cards.

Ectogenesis has been addressed in much scientific philosophical writing (Harris 1998; Singer and Wells 1984; Strong 2002), as well as in popular media. As I pointed out in the previous chapter, while some medical sources have avoided discussing this topic, others chose to address the advent of the artificial womb as a matter of fact (Ber 2000). Further advancements in fetal care research have provoked novel academic discussion (see Chap. 10). The artificial womb, however, is not exactly welcomed, with most countries banning research on human embryos beyond day 14. Canada has explicitly prohibited any research that is designed to add to the knowledge about ectogenesis (Final Report of the Royal Commission on New Reproductive Technologies 1993). Nonetheless, since prematurely born babies spend less time in

A version of this chapter was published in the Cambridge Quarterly of Healthcare Ethics: Simonstein, F. and Mashiach Eizenberg, M. (2009). The Artificial Womb: A Pilot Study Considering People's Views on the Artificial Womb and Ectogenesis in Israel. Cambridge Quarterly of Healthcare Ethics, 18(1): 87–94.

a woman's womb, the question of the minimum amount of time an embryo "should" spend in a woman's womb (nine months? six? five? two days?), and why, cannot be easily answered.

As I observed in the previous chapter, if proved one day to be safe, the solution of ectogenesis might avoid the need for a surrogate among women who want a biological baby but lack a womb (for any reason); and possibly also for homosexual male couples. The idea might also appeal to women who may need IVF to reproduce, potentially saving them time, pain, depression, and endless frustration (when embryos fail to implant, for instance). Moreover, the AW may prevent damage to women's health since it may avoid short- and/or long-term negative effects either during or after a pregnancy (Altman et al. 2006; Ayers et al. 2006; Russell et al. 1996).[1] For although pregnancy is not considered an illness (Cook et al. 2003), it is not exactly a health enterprise, either, and without proper medical care, can be deadly.[1]

Even more contentious, as many authors have pointed out, is that ectogenesis may finally achieve equality for women; since a woman who wants a child might not necessarily be forced to hinder her career progression because of a pregnancy. Although gender inequality is mainly a result of childcare and a vast range of other gender-related issues, and not necessarily because of the pregnancy itself, its roots may be found in the fact that women (unlike men) are the ones who bear the child and, therefore, must slow down. For some women, the option of a genuine choice of whether to bear the child (or not), in order to become a parent, could be of value (see also Chap. 10).

These issues are highly controversial and present in academic discussion, but little is known about the views of the general public on these topics. The aim of this study, therefore, was to start to fill this gap: Its purpose was to explore the attitudes of Israeli lay people—in a pro-natalistic country that has eagerly adopted IVF—toward the advent of the AW. In the context of womb politics, awareness of people's views on this topic could be useful for further discussion about the present ethical and legal situation and developing appropriate legislation. Therefore, similar studies may also develop in other countries. Although ectogenesis and the artificial womb are not the same (as I noted in the previous chapter, ectogenesis is the process and the artificial womb is the tool), also in this chapter I use these expressions interchangeably.

11.1 Research Methods

The study included 216 subjects aged over 21 who answered a structured self-report questionnaire. The questionnaire was divided into two sections: The first part addressed the respondent's personal data (such as gender, age, family status, number of children, profession). The second part targeted the respondent's views regarding the AW. This part included 12 statements ranked on a Likert scale between 1 =

---

[1] This list is not exhaustive. See also "Pregnancy Hazards" in the previous chapter.

strongly disagree and 5 = strongly agree. Half of the statements were negative and the other half were positive. The "position score" was calculated as the average of all the respondent's answers (after appropriate reversal of the scale for the negative statements). A score close to 1 determined a strong negative position, indicating that the respondent was strongly against the AW. A score close to 5 expressed a positive stance, indicating that the respondent strongly agreed with this development. The internal consistency (Cronbach's alpha) of the position score was 0.899. The sample in this survey was obtained by a snowball method (i.e., referrals by respondents, which generated additional subjects). One obvious limitation of this mode of sampling is that it may affect the representative nature of the sample. However, although not representative (there were fewer men than women), the sample in this study included different sections of the Israeli population.

Table 11.1 shows that the percentage of women in this survey was three times higher than the percentage of men, which may suggest that men would be less responsive to this questionnaire than women. The majority of respondents in this survey were aged 31–51, but nearly one third of the sample were younger than 31. The sample also included a smaller proportion of respondents who were above the age of 51.

Most subjects were married, nearly one third were single, and a small number were divorced or widowed. The majority had from one to three children, a small proportion had more than four children, and one third had none. Most of the subjects in this study were Jewish, but there was a good representation of non-Jews (Christians, Muslims, and Druze), as well. While most of the respondents were secular, there was also a good percentage of those who identified themselves as "traditional," and a smaller percentage reported being religious to varying degrees. The majority were born in Israel, but there was also a fair representation of immigrants. An equal percentage of respondents had received either an academic or vocational education, while a smaller fraction had received only 12 years of schooling.

11.2 Results

While people's attitudes toward the AW were explored through randomly ordered statements in the questionnaire, in this report, the responses were grouped in four distinctive categories for better clarity. The first group contained statements reflecting a general position towards the AW; the second related to statements about possible uses of the artificial womb, and the third category included possible uses of the artificial womb specifically related to women's reproductive tasks. In addition, the questionnaire examined the extent to which, in two given situations, the respondent would use the AW in practice: in order to save their own fetus and/or to avoid a pregnancy (Table 11.2).

Table 11.2 shows that just 10.2% of all the respondents thought that the artificial womb should not be developed under any circumstances; by contrast, 76.8% of all respondents were against this statement. Although 47.2% of all respondents agreed

Table 11.1 Personal characteristics of the subjects

	Response	Percentage (%)	Mean ± (SD)
Gender			
Man	51	24	
Woman	165	76	
Age			35.8 ± (9.94)
21–30	68	31.60	
31–50	131	61	
51 and older	16	7.40	
Family status			
Single	69	31.90	
Married	138	63.90	
Divorced or widowed	9	4.20	
Children			1.61 ± (1.54)
0	82	38.70	
1–3	108	51.00	
4 or more	22	10.30	
Religion			
Jewish	156	72.60	
Christian, Muslim, or Druze	68	27.40	
Religiosity			
Religious	20	9.30	
Traditional	59	27.30	
Secular	137	63.40	
Origin			
Native Israeli	155	72	
Immigrant	59	28	
Education			
High school	22	10	
Vocational training	97	45	
Academic	96	45	

that the development of a fetus in AWs is against human nature, a majority of 57.9% disagreed with the statement that the development of a fetus in AW is against human dignity. Of all respondents, 65% agreed that it is important to develop the artificial womb to save the lives of premature fetuses and 53% agreed that its development is important for research to improve the effectiveness of IVF. Nearly 43% of the respondents agreed that it is important to develop the artificial womb to avoid the

Table 11.2 Attitudes toward the artificial womb (AW) proportions (%) of responses (N = 216)

Item		Proportions (%) of responses			
		Disagree	Partly agree	Agree	Missing
General position toward the AW	The AW should not be developed under any circumstances	76.8	11.6	10.2	1.4
	The development of a fetus in the AW is against human nature	35.2	16.7	47.2	0.9
	The development of a fetus in the AW is against human dignity	57.9	21.3	19.9	0.9
Possible uses of AW	It is important to develop the AW to save premature babies	18.5	15.7	65.3	0.5
	It is important to develop the AW for research to improve IVF effectiveness	22.2	22.7	53.2	1.9
	It is important to develop the AW to avoid the need for surrogates	36.6	19.9	42.6	0.9
	It is important to develop the AW for women who do not have a womb	9.7	15.3	74.5	0.5
Possible uses of the AW (related to women's challenging reproductive tasks)	Women should not be allowed to have the choice of using the AW	36.7	11.1	50.9	1.4
	It is important to develop the AW to ease women's tasks in society	67.9	18.9	13.0	0.9
	It is important to develop the AW to enable women to choose how to have children	59.3	13.0	26.4	1.4
Possible use of the AW by the respondent	I would use the AW (for myself or for my partner) to avoid a pregnancy	86.5	3.2	7.8	2.3
	I would use the AW to save my fetus if it was in danger	15.8	13.0	71.3	0.0

need for surrogates; and notably, a large majority—74.5%—thought that its development is important for women who do not have a womb. The majority of respondents, 71.3%, thought they would use an AW to save their own fetus. Contrary to this relatively large percentage of positive views towards the AW, when women's challenging reproductive tasks were at the center of the statements, respondents' views became less receptive: nearly 51% thought that women should not have the opportunity of choosing freely to use the artificial womb. Regarding the statement that it is not important to develop the AW so that women can choose how to give birth, 59% of respondents agreed, and 67.9% thought that it is not important to develop the artificial womb to ease women's reproductive tasks. Accordingly, a large majority, 87% of the respondents, thought that they would not use the AW to avoid a pregnancy.

We further analyzed the link between sociodemographic data and people's attitudes toward the advent of the AW. Table 11.3 presents an analysis of the correlation between people's sociodemographic backgrounds and their views. It shows that men and single people of both genders had a significantly more positive approach toward the AW. There was a negative correlation between the number of children and attitude toward the AW, i.e., respondents with fewer children had more positive attitudes. Jewish respondents were significantly more positive toward the development of the AW than non-Jewish respondents. A negative correlation was found also between the level of reported religiosity and the acceptance of AW, i.e., secular people were more positive toward the artificial womb. Finally, there was a significant difference between the mean attitudes toward the AW according to education level. Respondents with an academic degree were more positive toward this development.

Table 11.3 Relationship between sociodemographic background and attitude toward the AW (mean attitude index)

Variable		N	Mean	Standard deviation	t-test	Correlation
Gender	Woman	165	3.00	0.85	$t(214) = 4.87**$	
	Man	51	3.67	0.83		
Family status	Single	69	3.38	0.90	$t(205) = 2.56*$	
	Married	138	3.05	0.88		
Religion	Jewish	156	3.31	0.85	$t(205) = 4.34**$	
	Not Jewish	59	2.75	0.82		
Education	Academic	96	3.30	0.91	$t(213) = 2.00*$	
	High school	119	3.06	0.86		
Age		215				$r = 0.032$
Children		215				$r = -0.278**$
Religiosity		216				$r = -0.364**$

Significance level: $*P < 0.05$, $**P < 0.001$

11.3 Discussion

As observed also in Chap. 10 of this book, following Firestone's stand on ectogenesis (Firestone 2003 [1970]), Smajdor suggested that instead of placing the burden on women to have children when it suits the interest of society rather than the interests of individual women, society could advance "technical alternatives," such as artificial wombs. Smajdor challenges her readers with the following question:

> You, the reader, from behind the veil of ignorance (Smajdor refers here to John Rawls' thought experiment (Rawls 1971)) are asked whether you would prefer to be born into society A, where women bear all the risks and burdens of gestation and childbirth, as they do now, or society B, where ectogenesis has been perfected and is routinely used. You do not know whether you will be born as a man or a woman. Which would you choose? (Smajdor 2007)

The survey above echoes Smajdor's hypothetical question. Yet, contrary to her implicit hope that people would choose society B, the majority of respondents in this study chose to be born into society A. Moreover, paradoxically, perhaps, more women than men in this survey would prefer to bear all the risks, as well as the burdens of gestation and childbirth traditionally associated with womanhood. Nevertheless, this study suggests that, in general, people's attitudes toward AWs are not as negative as might be expected.

While people in this survey were markedly against using AW for ectogenesis, the majority did not think that the artificial womb should not be developed under any circumstances. Most of the respondents agreed that the AW is not natural for human beings; however, a large proportion disagreed with the statement that the AW is against human dignity. Remarkably, three out of four people in this survey accepted the idea that AWs could resolve the problem of childlessness for women who do not have a womb. Respondents also attributed significant value to the development of the AW to save the lives of premature fetuses and for IVF research. Most tellingly, perhaps, the majority of people in this survey thought that they would use AWs to save the life of their own fetus, if it were in danger. This position reflects the societal pressure toward the development of the AW.

In sharp contrast to this view, however, when the statements centered on the idea of easing women's "natural" reproductive roles, the AW was considered unacceptable. Most of the respondents disagreed with the idea that it may be important to develop AWs to give women an alternative means of having children. Most also disagreed with the notion that women could be allowed to choose AWs freely. Most of the respondents did not accept the statement that it is important to develop AWs to make women's lives easier. In short, people's acceptance of AWs centered neither on reducing women's challenging reproductive tasks nor on providing women with the option of having a real choice in reproductive matters. In accordance with that, most people in this survey thought that they would not use an AW to avoid a pregnancy. It is noteworthy that the mean attitude of men in this survey was significantly more positive toward AWs (although fewer men than women participated). Further analysis of gendered positions revealed also that a lower percentage of women than men approved of the idea that AWs could alleviate women's reproductive tasks.

While 87% of the women in this survey (N = 165) agreed with the statement that pregnancy and childbirth are not healthy for a woman's body, 92% of the women thought that pregnancy is not a disease. Most of the women, 89%, agreed that pregnancy and childbirth are important experiences for womanhood. We also asked the women who already had children (N = 105) to mark, on a scale of 1–10, the degree of difficulty they had experienced during pregnancy and childbirth (1 = very easy; 10 = very difficult). Of the women who had children, 39% ranked the experience of pregnancy as very difficult (8–10 on the scale) and 44% reported childbirth as a very difficult experience.

Nonetheless, we did not find a significant link between the general position toward the AW and the difficulty of pregnancy and childbirth. This was despite the positive correlation between the difficulty that a woman experienced during the pregnancy and her willingness to use the AW to avoid a pregnancy ($p < 0.05$). The fact that women were significantly less receptive toward AWs in this study is hardly surprising because in Israel (for religious and demographic reasons), there is strong societal conditioning of girls toward motherhood. As noted also in Chap. 3 of this book, Israeli girls (regardless of religion) learn from early childhood that infertility is a curse (Kahn 2000). Even secular, well-educated, and wealthy women in Israeli society believe that it is their duty to have children (Remennick 2000). Accordingly, the majority of women in this survey agreed with the statement that pregnancy and childbirth are key experiences for a woman.

Interestingly, however, this endorsement of womanhood was negatively correlated with age. A larger number of older women disagreed with this statement, suggesting that life experience, beyond the reproductive years, plays a role in women's perspective of womanhood. Although most people in this survey were against using AWs to avoid a pregnancy, there was, nevertheless, a positive correlation between the general attitude toward the development of AWs and the respondent's level of secularity and education. Thus, in this study, secular and well-educated people were more receptive toward AWs. The findings suggest that positive developments in this technology could enhance people's receptiveness toward the AW in Israel. However, it is difficult to predict how people will react when AW technology becomes fully developed and safe (A Report of the President's Council on Bioethics 2004).

11.4   Some Lessons Learned from IVF

Back in the early seventies, IVF was considered by some as repulsive and as a monstrosity. If IVF were to be allowed, all stabilizing threads would unravel, threatening "the very fabric of civilization:"

> Marriage, fidelity, the essence of family; the sense of who we are and where we're headed; what it means to be human, connected, normal, acceptable; that it will threaten our ideas about love, sex, and nurturance. (Marantz-Henig 2004)

The same words apply now to ectogenesis. However, as noted also in Chaps. 7 and 8, IVF has become "routine." It is covered by medical insurance plans and has been used by infertile couples around the world. In 2018, according to a report by the European Society of Human Reproduction and Embryology (ESHRE), more than 8 million babies had already been born with the aid of IVF.[2] Thus, the apocalyptic predictions about IVF had not been realized. At the time, however, IVF caused many to consider the possibilities of future ill-use and the method was far from acceptable. The impression was that it might never become generally tolerated—much less embraced. Nevertheless, soon after the first successful birth of "test-tube baby" Louise Brown, in 1978, a poll showed that 60% of Americans thought that IVF should be available for anyone who needed and wanted it.

Will this be the case with ectogenesis as well? The answer is difficult to predict, but as the survey reported in this chapter suggests, people may accept the use of artificial wombs to solve reproductive problems. The use of ectogenesis to alleviate women's role in reproduction is not acceptable according to this survey. However, shortly after the birth of Louise Brown, a committee of the National Academy of Sciences observed, in its Report Assessing Biomedical Technologies, that the initial reaction to a given use of a technology might be very different from later reactions, should that technology become familiar over years of general use. Attitudes, the report said, have a habit of changing; people may think and feel differently in the future about marriage, procreation, or kinship, and the biological family. It is, therefore, risky to predict how people might react to some of the future technological prospects. As Henig observes:

> [P]eople have felt revulsion towards most emerging technologies, especially those that mimic functions we take to be central to our definitions of life and death, and that make us unique and human. These technologies at first often seem gruesome or barbaric in prospect, filled with technical impossibilities or ethical conundrums. (Marantz-Henig 2004)

Marantz-Henig also reminds us that blood transfusion, organ transplantation, mechanical respirators, and artificial insemination were all greeted with suspicion; but as soon as these procedures were performed successfully several times, the objections faded away. Nevertheless, it is essential to acknowledge and respect the views of the population. Singer, for example, suggested that AWs could resolve the outcry against abortions (i.e., aborted fetuses could continue their lives in AWs) (Singer and Wells 1984). Contrary to Singer's idea, however, a study targeting women who had had abortions revealed that women who wished to terminate a pregnancy were not necessarily in favor of having their aborted fetuses kept alive (Cannold 2000).

11.5 Conclusions

In the present survey, most people found the use of AWs to solve reproductive problems to be an acceptable idea, but only a small fraction of the respondents said they would be willing to use an AW to avoid a pregnancy—but this could still amount to a significant number of people in the population. Moreover, strong views against technologies involving interventions on human beings have a tendency to change (as has happened with IVF, for example), after a novel procedure is successful.

Further developments in the AW might prove that ectogenesis could become as safe as (or even safer?) than a natural pregnancy for both parties involved: the fetus, which is the priority today, *and* his or her mother. However, as noted in the previous chapter, ethical and legal conundrums concerning the present legislation in most countries would be huge.

In the context of womb politics, research addressing the population's views (in Israel and in other parts of the globe) on the advent of AWs is essential. Additional study, in-depth analysis, and a broader discussion on ectogenesis, not only by ethicists, legal advisers, and politicians, but also among the wider public— while processing new improvements—is necessary also for developing appropriate legislation.

Notes

(1) http://www.who.int/pmnch/en/. Accessed 2 Apr 2021.
(2) https://www.sciencedaily.com/releases/2018/07/180703084127.htm. Accessed 2 Apr 2021.

References

A Report of the President's Council on Bioethics. 2004. *Reproduction and Responsibility. The Regulation of New Biotechnologies.* Washington, DC. http://www.bioethics.gov.

Altman, D., et al. 2006. Risk of Urinary Incontinence After Childbirth: A 10-Year Prospective Cohort Study. *Obstetrics & Gynecology* 108: 873–878.

Ayers, S., A. Eagle, and H. Waring. 2006. The Effects of Childbirth-Related Post-Traumatic Stress Disorder on Women and Their Relationships: A Qualitative Study Psychology. *Health and Medicine* 11: 389–398.

Ber, R. 2000. Ethical Issues in Gestational Surrogacy. *Theoretical Medicine and Bioethics* 21: 153–169.

Cannold, L. 2000. *The Abortion Myth: Feminism, Morality, and the Hard Choices Women Make.* Hannover, NH: University Press of New England.

Cook, R., B.M. Dickens, and M.F. Fathalla. 2003. *Reproductive Health and Human Rights.* New York: Oxford University Press.

Final Report of the Royal Commission on New Reproductive Technologies. 1993. *Minister of Government Services, Canada.* Ottawa: Canada Communications Group.

Firestone, S. 2003 [1970]. *The Dialectic of Sex: The Case for Feminist Revolution*, 3rd ed. New York: Farrar, Straus and Giroux.

Harris, J. 1998. *Clones, Genes and Immortality.* Oxford: Oxford University Press.

Henig, R. Marantz. 2004. *Pandora's Baby.* New York: Houghton Mifflin.

Kahn, S.M. 2000. *Reproducing Jews. A Cultural Account of Assisted Conception in Israel Durham.* North Carolina: Duke University Press.

Kuperman, T., D. Elad, D. Grisaru, et al. 2020. Tissue-Engineered Multi-Cellular Models of the Uterine Wall. *Biomechanics and Modeling in Mechanobiology* 19: 1629–1639.

Partridge, E.A., M.G. Davey, M.A. Hornick, and A.W. Flake. 2017. An EXTrauterine Environment for Neonatal Development: EXTENDING Fetal Physiology Beyond the Womb. *Seminars in Fetal and Neonatal Medicine* 22 (6): 404–409.

Rawls, J. 1971. *A Theory of Justice*. Cambridge: Cambridge University Press.

Remennick, L. 2000. Childless in the Land of Imperative Motherhood: Stigma and Coping Among Infertile Israeli Women. *Sex Roles* 43: 821–824.

Russell, R., R. Dundas, and F. Reynolds. 1996. Long Term Backache After Childbirth: Prospective Search for Causative Factors. *BMJ* 312: 1384–1388.

Simonstein, F. 2006. Artificial Reproduction Technologies—All the Way to the Artificial Womb? *Philosophy of Medicine and Health Care* 9: 359–365.

Singer, P., and D. Wells. 1984. *The Reproduction Revolution: New Ways to Making Babies*. Oxford: Oxford University Press.

Smajdor, A. 2007. The Moral Imperative for Ectogenesis. *Cambridge Quarterly of Healthcare Ethics* 16: 336–345.

Strong, C. 2002. Overview: A Framework for Reproductive Ethics. In *Ethical Issues in Maternal-Fetal Medicine*, ed. Dona L. Dickenson. Cambridge: Cambridge University Press.

Conclusions

Womb Politics entails having power over the womb—in fact, over people who possess one. This theme of power over the womb is a thread running through all of the issues discussed in this book. This volume covers an extensive terrain, with the aim of presenting a broader picture of the politics of the womb (i.e., the social demands over women's role in human reproduction). Hence its examination of topics and disciplines that are usually discussed separately. In this book, I have explored gendered issues, demographic needs, requests, and commands that have laid down rules about the womb since biblical times. I have examined the advent of the pill, decriminalization of contraception in the 1960s, and have explored the struggle for lawful abortions around the world that is still ongoing in the twenty-first century.[1] I looked at assisted reproduction technologies (ARTS) that developed in the last decade of the twentieth century, pointing to its uses and possible abuses. Finally, I explored reprogenetics and the potential demand for all women to reproduce via IVF, to allow genetically enhanced future generations. Such a demand may advance the advent of the artificial womb (AW).

Chapter 2 explored the notions of sex and gender. It showed that whereas a person's sex—the attributes that distinguish males from females—is a biological determinant, gender—or the behavior and roles that a person experiences and expresses—are not. Gender remains a social construct in which masculinity and femininity are a set of habits, traditions, and beliefs woven deeply as social behaviors in which we are schooled from birth by parents, friends, and teachers. We are taught that some gendered lifestyle choices are appropriate for us, while others are not. Thus, we become "women" and "men" by playing a predetermined role imposed by society. Gendered roles have been biased, however, favoring men throughout human history. Theories explaining why patriarchal rules developed in all human societies remain

---

[1] At the time of finalizing this book (May 2022) there is a US Supreme Court draft opinion to overturn Roe v. Wade. https://www.politico.com/news/2022/05/02/supreme-court-abortion-draft-opinion-00029473.

F. Simonstein, *Womb Politics: A Short History of the Future of Human Reproduction*, The International Library of Bioethics 99, https://doi.org/10.1007/978-3-031-11654-4

unsatisfactory. Nevertheless, women's dependence on men because of the daily need for survival after giving birth played a role.

The Feminist Movement that developed in the nineteenth century, following human rights and egalitarian ideals, started (at last) to demand rights and equality for women. Women's lot has improved; but disparities that favor men at the top remain. While more girls than boys are doing better at school, college, and university, women disappear further up the ladder, and those who make it to the top of their careers are the exceptions. What happens in the gap between the first steps of a successful woman's career and her advance up the ladder toward the top is having babies and raising children, becoming stranded in the so-called "motherhood penalty." Presently, motherhood is considered a woman's choice. But is it really a choice? The most powerful gender imperative is that motherhood is not only a woman's capability—by possessing a womb—but also her duty. And the most influential and prevailing source of this belief is the Bible.

Chapter 3 focused on the Bible. "Be fertile and replenish the earth" is the first commandment in the Bible, preceding the Ten Commands; and is the first written policy involving the womb. While God had ordered humans to be fruitful, barrenness—the worst curse for a woman according to the Bible—remains a central topic. Barrenness and God's miraculous intervention of opening wombs return, in the Bible, again and again. Fertility in the Bible is so crucial that the four matriarchs happen to be barren. They conceive only after God lifts the curse that "closed" their wombs. According to the Bible, childlessness for a woman is worse than death; so much so that it is even acceptable to practice prostitution and deception in order to conceive.

Scholars have considered the stories in the book of Genesis as an etiologic explanation of the world. However, the Bible's vigorous promotion of reproduction seems odd, since children usually arrive naturally after heterosexual intercourse. And it is unlikely that people in ancient times abstained from heterosexual activity. In those days, many newborns did not survive for numerous reasons, including that women had to abandon them for their own survival. Aiming at better demographic outcomes for political reasons, powerful new biblical doctrines developed. To persuade people to "buy" the new ideas—according to present notions of marketing—the writers of the Bible had to promote them effectively. Hence the repetitive biblical teaching that a woman's role is to be with child. She is the recipient who perpetuates her man's seed.

Evidently, the marketing strategy of fertility in the Bible has been successful, since more than two millennia later, in the twenty-first century, women are still internalizing this role. "Be fertile" has remained a powerful commandment in cultures based on the three monotheist religions and continues to dictate women's lives until today. To be a woman with child remains—explicitly and implicitly—a social directive. Childless women are—supposed to be—miserable; and pitied. So much so that, in the twenty-first century, a woman's "destiny" may still rely on her ability to reproduce. For many women, infertility continues to be an insufferable state. In present times, demographic whims addressing the womb persist.

Chapter 4 explored demography, which relates to the scientific study of population, the "numbering of the people." Current demography tries to understand population change in response to changes in fertility, mortality, and migration. While mortality is a predetermined figure (inevitably, we all die), fertility is not. Demographers have observed that fertility responds to biology, economics, and technology, but it is commonly acknowledged that ideational factors of individual preferences and social norms are the primary determinants of the timing and rate of childbearing. Women's education has emerged as a central predictor of fertility decline, and similarities across sites suggest that there are common elements in how education drives demographic transitions cross-culturally. Nevertheless, the differences suggest that local socioecologies also play an important role in the relationship between education and fertility decline. According to demographers, deeper analysis of how human culture, human ecology, and the human environment coevolve is necessary for understanding historical and present dynamics, and for predicting future trends: to plan directly and act accordingly, to reach optimal solutions.

Demographic planning, directions, and actions obviously target the womb. Indeed, some current political leaders (e.g., Russian President Putin, Turkish President Erdoğan, and Brazilian President Bolsonaro) see population growth as a national imperative and high fertility as "a female duty." Pope Francis also stated that "opting not to have children is a 'selfish choice.'" On the other hand, the right of couples to determine the number and spacing of their children is, currently, almost universally endorsed, whereas the possibility of coercive family planning is almost as widely condemned. But this was not the case until the second half of the twentieth century.

Chapter 5 examined the advent of the pill in the 1960s, the influential development that affected actual demography and family planning and, most importantly, enormously improved women's lives. Today, women who are young—and not so young—may be unaware of the enormous struggle that developing the pill entailed. In the third decade of the twenty-first century, it is no easy task to appreciate the huge obstacles that faced Margaret Sanger, Katharine McCormick, Gregory Pincus, and John Rock, 70 years ago, to make the pill available for women. Sanger and McCormick, the two "mothers" of the pill, insisted that female control of contraception was a prerequisite for women's emancipation. Since women disproportionately bore the burden of pregnancy and childrearing, they believed that women should have a contraceptive that they alone controlled. They foresaw birth control as helping women to overcome some of the fundamental inequalities of being women, that it would liberate them to seek further education, pursue more gainful employment, and raise healthier and better-educated children. To achieve their goal, they enlisted the help of scientist Gregory Pincus who enrolled a Catholic physician, John Rock, in their struggle.

Sanger used the euphemism of family planning to make the idea of contraception more palatable to politicians and policy makers. Today, the WHO—but not only the WHO—uses these terms interchangeably and promotes contraception and family planning worldwide. In creating the pill, Sanger and McCormick—the two women activists—ushered in what one historian called "the contraceptive mentality"—the belief in a woman's right to control her own fertility. The pill liberated many women, allowing them to postpone or prevent motherhood in favor of other opportunities, such as higher education and employment. This is one reason why it is often viewed as a key milestone for women's rights, and one of the greatest inventions of the twentieth century. However, women's struggle in the abortion camp is a different story.

Chapter 6 explored the abortion wars, still fought by women (and men) around the world. Conceiving a child is a happy event. However, if the pregnancy is not wanted, the woman in question can experience it as terrifying. Many women in this situation feel being trapped by their own bodies. And although induced abortion is not exactly a favorite small-talk topic among women who have had one, approximately 56 million induced abortions are performed worldwide each year. Nevertheless, in addition to the physical and mental ordeal of abortion, women, almost everywhere, are not allowed to decide what to do with their own bodies. In more than 92% of all countries, women must receive permission from the state to abort legally. In different countries globally, abortion is either illegal altogether, illegal but permitted in some cases, or legal. Even if abortion in a particular country is permitted, access can be restricted by gestational age, third-party authorization mandates, and an assortment of service-delivery requirements.

Among the countries with legal abortion is the United States, where it was legalized in 1973 under the right of privacy by the ruling in the Roe v. Wade case. Even then, "the interest of the state" may overrule the interest of the woman to end the pregnancy: states could regulate and even prohibit abortions, balancing between a woman's right to privacy and the state's interests. Thus, even in Roe v. Wade, the state continued to own women's bodies.

The Global Gag Rule (GGR) prohibits NGOs who receive U.S. global health assistance from providing legal abortion services or referrals, while also barring advocacy for abortion law reform—even when funded independently by the NGO. In January 2022, President Joseph Biden rescinded the GGR. However, when the Republicans regain power, they will most probably reinstate it. Anyway, in the two most-restrictive categories of countries, abortions occur as frequently as in the least-restrictive category. Highly restrictive laws do not eliminate the practice of abortion but make those that do occur more likely to be unsafe. According to the Guttmacher Institute, the situation may be improving, as some countries may now allow abortion in more cases. However, the Guttmacher Institute also recommends expanding the legal grounds, obtaining safer abortions for more women. It is horrifying that there are about 1 billion women, living almost everywhere in the world, who still need permission to have an abortion. And the main and very basic question remains: If the pregnancy is unwanted, why on earth should women have to ask permission from "the state"—or from anyone—to terminate it. This notwithstanding, helping women to become pregnant in the first place has been welcomed, celebrated, and copiously funded.

Chapter 7 explored assisted reproduction: how lab-produced embryos and pregnancies achieved by medical intervention have changed our perception of human reproduction, further challenging women's role in their reproductive tasks. In this chapter, I presented the politics of IVF, of which many women—and men—remain unaware. IVF was developed during a time when women were becoming liberated from unwanted pregnancies, with the development of the pill and the legalization of abortion. Nonetheless, stories of infertile women "desperately" wanting children and pursuing IVF brought back the idealization of a maternal vocation that every "normal" woman must have. Infertile women wanting children and undergoing IVF became publicly applauded.

More than four decades have passed since the first child was born as a result of IVF in 1978; and despite much initial resistance by the medical community and by society, IVF has become the first rather than the last option for treating infertility. Even so, my contention is that the development of IVF has been the largest experiment ever performed on human subjects. And it seems to have remained experimental. Despite the enormous increase in treatment of infertility with IVF, the overall success rate with IVF cycles has remained low. Less than 50% of women will achieve a pregnancy with IVF, and even fewer will get a take-home baby. In addition, IVF is riskier than a natural pregnancy, and the long-term dangers remain unclear. Nevertheless, IVF is advertised in an utterly optimistic and misleading manner. Indeed, IVF has developed a Teflon reputation, being promoted by a thriving industry.

IVF has further medicalized and technologized reproduction, and whereas this development has increased procreative liberties for some, IVF has also reduced the freedom of others. In developed societies, women might feel free to (not) commit themselves to IVF, if they (do not) want to. But even in these countries, since the procedure exists, women may still feel obligated to use it. The pressure on women to reproduce, marketed as "this is what women do; and want," persists. It has been suggested that, rather than IVF, it is the societal factors coercing women to reproduce that should be addressed. However, the question of whether women are coerced into IVF has remained largely unanswered. In pronatalist societies, women do not seem to have much hope of escaping from IVF, especially if it is funded by the state.

Chapter 8 presented the use—and misuse—of IVF in Israel, a developed country with a pronatalist society. Israel has an open-ended policy of IVF of up to two children in a relationship, even if the woman already has children. Israel may be a special case, but its IVF policy is considered the North Star for supplying IVF, worldwide. This policy is widely considered as very generous and consistent with women's "needs" and "rights."

At first sight, the Israeli IVF policy might be taken as an example to be followed worldwide, as it seems to be a win-win situation, with all the stakeholders benefiting equally under the ultra-permissive policy. However, a closer examination suggests that this may not be the case. Israeli women embark on very lengthy IVF treatment and, in too many cases, end up worse off. Low-cost treatment with IVF may help some women but may become a "perseverance trap" for others. The "culture of perseverance" with IVF in Israel has been on the rise—against the odds and despite other health hazards.

In a retrospective analysis of IVF in two Israeli clinics, we found the open-ended IVF policy to be ineffective. For women under 40, the data showed that the probability of having a child after seven IVF attempts is zero. Women over 40 reach zero probability after four cycles with IVF. The procedure is now considered "routine," but remains highly ineffective as each IVF cycle has an average of 83–85% failure and long-term treatment side effects are, so far, unknown. The results of this research reveal the inadequacy of the unlimited IVF rounds policy. We recommended a systematic long-term assessment of the health and welfare of women after IVF—especially after prolonged treatment.

During (and before) the 1970s, IVF began as an experiment on childless women, sometimes even without their knowledge. They were (cheap) guinea pigs. Today, women do sign an informed consent form; but it is questionable how genuinely informed they are, as misleading information about IVF generally gets the upper hand. In fact, the informed consent document is worded to ensure the clinic and its physicians full protection from any charges. We suggested that further *independent* research, both retrospective and prospective, is needed to develop a truly informed policy for IVF in Israel and worldwide, which could assist patients' (women's) needs and also protect their health. As a result, a cautionary guideline was issued in Israel, but this guideline is not binding; hence the continuing unlimited policy regarding IVF.

In the context of womb politics, the chapters on IVF presented a perspective of the various politics that reign over the womb. Nevertheless, some compare the birth of the first IVF baby, in 1978, with the technological advance of humans walking on the moon. Yet the low efficacy of any single IVF cycle remains questionable. We may assume that not many (or no?) men would submit themselves to a non-lifesaving, demanding, and risky medical procedure that has an 80% failure rate per cycle—a result that has remained constant for two decades. In the not too distant future, however, all women—not only those experiencing infertility—may find themselves facing further reproductive risks and experimentation with the development of reprogenetics, the merging of molecular genetics and IVF.

Chapter 9 focused on reprogenetics. It connected the dots of an elusive picture: from a growing mature and aging population in chronic ill health and health care allocation to genetic editing of the germline as a possible solution. Editing the germline to improve the health of future generations may coincide with public health goals; it may improve the health of individuals and communities, and, if successful, may be seen as being for the public good. However, enhancing future generations will require PGD and IVF.

This begs the question of whether all women might have to conceive with IVF. Remarkably, the proponents of an enhancing scenario have not discussed the necessary involvement of women. The present discourse on moral obligations to future generations, although not referring to women, seems to imply that women might be required, morally, if not legally, to reproduce with IVF. Enhancing evolution with gene editing of the germline would be a gendered project. Therefore, questions about women's role in this scenario must be addressed. Moreover, the idea of and the reasons for enhancing evolution in a reprogenic context might *invite* the advent of the artificial womb.

Chapter 10 focused on the advent of the artificial womb and ectogenesis. The AW has been the focus of arduous research and might become a reality sooner than we think, as developments in neonatal care, gynecology, embryology, computer science, and the human genome project are converging to this end. The latest developments show that improvements have been made both at the end and the beginning of gesta-tion (ectogestation and ectogenesis, respectively). Although a huge gap remains in between, the history of science has shown that impenetrable barriers are temporary. It is only a matter of time (and research) until someone—either intentionally or by chance—finds a way to overcome an obstacle. Despite the apparent existence of too many barriers in the case of the artificial womb, it would be naïve to suppose that this invention may develop differently than in past scientific breakthroughs.

Presently, the aims of research toward the AW are to improve neonatal care for very premature babies, to achieve better embryo implantation in IVF, and to grow tissues and organs in the lab for transplant. Remarkably, not included in AW research is the aim of relieving women of the "health hazards" and "discomforts" that they currently endure in reproduction. The romantic view of pregnancy and childbirth and the societal conditioning of women to have babies remain fully at work. For some women (and men), however, the option to have a genuine choice of whether (or not) to bear a child in order to become a parent could be of value. Ectogenesis also has the potential to challenge traditional patriarchal family structures and all other male-dominated structures (at work, in education and overall, culturally). Yet the challenges that ectogenesis may entail regarding present ethics and legislation are huge. A discussion on the AW and ectogenesis has started in academic circles; however, lay people's views on the advent of the AW and ectogenesis are largely unknown.

Chapter 11 presented a survey of lay people's attitudes toward the artificial womb and ectogenesis in Israel. In this survey, most people accepted the idea of using AWs to solve reproductive problems, but only a small fraction of the respondents said they would be willing to use AW to avoid a pregnancy. Nevertheless, even this small fraction could amount to a significant number of people in the population.

Strong views against technologies involving interventions with human beings have a tendency to change after a novel procedure is successful (as happened with IVF, for example). Further developments in the AW might prove that ectogenesis could become as safe as (or even safer?) than a natural pregnancy for both parties involved: the fetus, which is the priority today, *and* his or her mother. Additional study, in-depth analysis, and a broader discussion on ectogenesis, not only by ethicists, legal advisers, and politicians, but also among the wider public, is necessary for developing appropriate legislation.

Final Remark

Inequality between the genders (men and women) still exists in the twenty-first century. This is mainly because women carry pregnancies; and women remain the main careers of their children after they are born. Of course, this has to do with the female physiology, as so far, only women have wombs. Yet the decision to have children, how many, where, how, and why, is politically driven. Whether in the academic and governmental spheres, or among lay people (women and men), all must acknowledge that the unique organ with which women are born—or endowed—is not private. The womb has been and remains a public organ, politically ruled. The question remains as to whether it will be possible to disengage the womb from either bold or subtle political intervention in the future. The answer depends largely on our awareness of, and response to, womb politics.

Index